His Hand Has Provided

*A Christian Cowboy's Guide
to Nutrition and Natural
Healing with Herbs*

CHRIS GUSSA

Disclaimer:
The mention of nutrition and herbs used as remedies is from the use of food and herbs from Traditional Folk Medicine and the use of food and herbs from Traditional Chinese Medicine. I am in no way intending to diagnose, treat or prevent any disease with any non- FDA approved drug. I am simply sharing information with anyone reading this book. I consider you all friends and therefore I am simply sharing what I know with friends.

ISBN: 1484975154
ISBN-13: 9781484975152

TABLE OF CONTENTS

TABLE OF CONTENTS

INTRODUCTION:

Not long ago I was at our Cowboy Church (Around Thanksgiving time) when our pastor asked us to share what we were thankful for as Christians. There were many great reasons to be thankful but as I thought about it I came to the conclusion that discerning (Or having the ability to plainly see what is right before God and what is not) was what I was thankful to have as a Christian. I guess I figured most of us had this.

As examples I thought about the media's politics and government's antichrist legislations allowing anything to be taught in schools except that awful "J word". Then I thought of how easily we can discern the evil of the absurd commercials that are pushing antidepressants and other dangerous drugs. This is for Christians? I thought. Surely, as Christians, we can all see through that.

Another thing was the overwhelming lack of desire of the general public to cook or prepare meals. This is evident in all the commercials advertising super processed unnatural food items based on convenience with absolutely no nutrition. How easy to discern this stuff as a Christian I thought!

I was just about to stand up and comment on these things when I realized, Wait a minute! The comments on drugs and lack of nutritional food would insult about 99% of the congregation because most of them were buying this entire media brain washing program hook line and sinker!

With God's help I stayed in my seat and prayed silently. What am I to do God? How can I approach this problem within your people without insulting them or with out sounding a bit crazy to them? Lord, please help. In essence, this is what finally convinced me to write this book.

I had already wanted to write a book on health for Christians just because I am convinced that God wants His people healthy but this was the straw that broke the camel's back. It should not be the Christians that suffer at the hands of Satan's lies. Christians should be leading the way to the truth of natural Godly health. Instead it looks like they are leading the way to an early grave.

All this does not mean we can't indulge in those wonderful Church parties centered on food sometimes. In fact it means, if we do it in God's name, and keep it healthy we can laugh heartier, stay awake longer, and enjoy these Christian fellowships even more as we rejoice in God's good health that He has provided.

PASTORS DON"T WORRY! You do not have to remove that fried chicken and apple pie from your list! We should; however make sure that what ever we eat is made from real food and not processed chemical ingredients we can't pronounce. Besides, fried chicken and apple pies made with the real stuff is five times as good tasting!

You will like finding out things like "REAL BUTTER is your friend" and "Wholesome organic raw sugar is not your enemy" (In moderation of course) You will also be glad to know that lots of organic beef and other animal products are really the kind of protein our bodies need most.

Yes, man (Adam) was originally created as a vegetarian but that was before the days of Noah's flood when we had that wonderful firmament around the earth. The huge vegetables and fruit that grew under that firmament were growing in a different barometric pressure caused by that same firmament. Because of this natural "barometric chamber" we know some men lived to be over 900 years old.

But let's face it, we sinned! It's done. God broke open His firmament and caused the waters to fall from the sky. This changed everything! Things would now ferment and rot. There was now pestilence. Man had been cursed by God for his sin. However that does not mean God doesn't still love us! Even with His curse came His blessings. He must chastise us at times but we must understand, He is our Father and will always love us.

Just because we can't live to be 900 years old anymore it does not mean we can't live a long healthy happy life and die peacefully at the age of 120. Most of us really could achieve this if we just listened to God and took only His wonderful bounty of whole food and medicine into our bodies as He has planned. So in short, His hand really HAS provided all that we need. He has given us all the earth to use wisely.

HOWEVER, when we take the individual molecules of God's creations from things such as petroleum and rearrange them into synthetic drugs and then enforce a federal law that says, "this is the only medicine doctors are allowed to administer or even refer to as REAL medicine" it becomes not only a deadly act of tyranny in America but it also mocks God.

So, you ask, what is going on? Why have our government and media teamed up to absolutely deny God and treat any thing good and wholesome as if it should be illegal? This causes many questions to suddenly demand an answer. Questions like:

Is it safe to eat anything from a store that is not labeled organic?

Why is there so much stuff sold as food that is not even real food?

Why is the media trying to shove this fake food down our throats?

Why do doctors keep pushing more and more dangerous drugs on us?

Is a hidden genocidal plan in the government behind all this?

How can we stay safe from poison disguised as food?

Can we use herbs as our medicine?

What is the FDA really all about?

Do those long jet contrails that never disappear and then turn into clouds have anything to do with this stuff?

What does God's word say about all this?

Well welcome to this book! I promise to do my best to answer these questions and many more. Sometimes the decisions that people must come to concerning all this "natural health verses a deadly toxic world" stuff can get a little heavy when we first realize what is going on. However God is in control and the fun part of this book is that we can always take a look at how the traditional cowboy would look at these situations. What would he do?

Chapter 1:
The Need for Nutrition

The Need for Nutrition in the Cowboy Churches

The modern cowboy of today is often the young man who is eager to get to work or try a new rope out or is ready to compete in a ranch rodeo event and just wants a quick "buzz" of energy from a fast meal of sugar doughnuts and coffee. And so all the cowboy churches tend to stock up on this type of thing for the ranch-rodeos and often fill up the snack table at the entrance of the churches every Sunday morning with this as well.

There always seems to be lots of packaged processed cookies, cakes and deserts full of deadly trans-fats and hydrogenated oils which are used for long shelf-life. Also, for some reason (As if it were a new "cowboy standard") you can always count on a great big jug of "Country Time Lemonade" next to the ice tea jug which often is made from a powdered tea mix as well.

Now God bless the hearts of those in the church who are only trying to "give 'em what they want" out of true Christian love. However we have to wake up and take a close and hard look at what we are doing to these cowboys and cowgirls. Most of all we have to look with compassion at their children who are really scarfing this stuff down! Lord, forgive us! (For we truly know not what we do)

In the next few pages you will read how even the FDA admitted the deadly poison known as benzene is produced in soft drinks like Country Time Lemonade. There is a whole heading coming up in this book on Country Time Lemonade and how thousands of deaths from many leukemia-type cancers have been a direct result. You will also see how and even get a glimpse of "why" the FDA together with the food and drug companies is successfully dumbing us down.

Folks, if I could cram all I am trying to say in one sentence it would be, **"Please only eat real food"** I can almost guarantee you will live 20 years longer if you do! That's twenty more years of serving Jesus on earth!

The way the FDA and media has brainwashed us, it is hard to see the difference between food and poison. We are lambs to the slaughter if we do not all wake up! Remember we are Christians and should be the ones setting the example of how to keep the temple of the Holy Spirit (which is our bodies) clean and healthy. *"Do you not know that your bodies are temples of the Holy Spirit, who is in you, whom you have received from God? You are not your own. You were bought at a price. Therefore honor God with your bodies"* 1st Corinthians 6:19-20

The easiest way to begin to understand what real food is and what is not is to first pray out loud to God almighty and ask Him to open your eyes that you may not be deceived by Satan and robbed of your daily bread. There is a lot we can take to our body's health from the way our Lord taught us to pray.

If you recall "The Lord's Prayer" than you will see we are first instructed to address the Father as Holy. Next we are instructed to pray for the Kingdom of Heaven to come and dwell with us on earth so that only God's will should be done.

The very first physical thing we are instructed to pray for is our daily bread! Now I don't know about you but I think that after asking our most Holy Father God for his will to be done on earth that He would not want us to eat some kind of corrupt processed food to poison the Holy temple of God! I am pretty sure this would this not be His will for us.

The point I am trying to make is when we ask for our daily bread, it is real wholesome God created food we are instructed to ask for and we should not ever let Satan replace it with anything else. We must expect only just what God said to pray for. We must be sure it is His bread made from God's real grains and not made from grain grown in Satan's genetically modified fields. If we pray for real wholesome food, then we will get it. God said so! It is an insult to God to accept anything else. (The frightening truth of how the Monsanto Company and the FDA are replacing America's food supply of God made grains and other crops with deadly genetically modified garbage is coming up soon in the next few chapters)

Remember we are both physical bodies and we are spiritual as well. The spiritual part of us is fed by staying in His will and reading His word. This is fairly easy to do when we truly love Jesus.

3

However keeping our bodies as a Holy Temple is not so easy to do today even when we do love Jesus.

It is so much easer to hit the drive-through fast food place and then have the nerve to ask God to "bless it to our bodies". We should have first had more respect for the Holy Temple and not let anything un-holy into the temple in the first place. Remember there is a big difference between food and "edible food-like substances" Daily bread means food as His hand has provided, being whole-some and above all, real food. Yes, the Bible says we can even eat food that was offered to idols if we bless it in His name but it surely does not ask us to seek it out and crave it. Also even food offered to Idols was still real food, not the processed garbage you see today.

The old saying amongst hopeful wives looking for a husband was, "The easiest way to a man's heart is through his stomach". Well it seems that Satan got hold of this saying and applied it to as, "The easiest way to destroy a man's heart is through his stomach"

Now after you have prayed, the first and best thing you can do in the physical is learn to read labels carefully. Don't worry; you don't need to know what those strange scientific chemical sound-ing names are! You just have to be sure you do NOT see them on the labels. The easiest short-cut is to only buy foods that have the name "Certified Organic" on them.

However when buying food (Not labeled Certified Organic) from a store the most important thing to look for is this: *If the in-gredients you are reading are anything other than animal (or natural animal product like eggs or honey) vegetable (or grain, flour, nuts or fruit etc.) or a mineral (like salt) than it is not a food. It is an edible, food-like substance.*

4

Put in basic scientific terms, *"There are, in fact, only three types of things on this earth that any substance can be made from. They are simply animal, vegetable and mineral."*

If what you are eating is simply one of these or any combination of these (In its natural form) than it could be considered safe and acceptable to our body as long as it was not a poisonous or otherwise unsafe natural substance.

If anything else shows up on the label it is typical of all non-organic "processed food"

What would an 1800's cowboy say about processed food?

Well, most likely he would say something like, *"What in the @&*# is that? Some kinda magic powder in a box? Your mixin' that poison powder in water and callin' it lemonade? Get that stuff away from me, I aint gettin' that no where near my mouth! Are you crazy?"*

One of the things the traditional cowboy had always taken pride in was the camp cook's ability to always cook great food while only carrying a few basic ingredients. These were flour, cornmeal, beans, rice, salt, spices, garlic, coffee and animal fat. Often, there was also sugar, honey, molasses and a few dried fruits like apples and apricots.

About the only kind of "processing" was beef jerky dried with salt and possibly some canned tomatoes. If you were really lucky you may have seen some canned peaches. You may have even seen some canned evaporated milk once in a while. This kind of "processing" for early canned goods required only heating and sealing and had nothing to do at all with the use of any chemicals. (Home canned foods from your garden are not considered "processed" just a naturally prepared great way to store food. It is a good safe practice and I encourage all of you who can to get into it)

Many times the camp cook's duties were also that of the "camp doctor". When this was the case., the camp cook's eye was always looking out for medicinal herbs growing that he knew could help heal wounds, stop infections, break fevers, ease pain, etc.

As for the meals, the camp cook's eyes were always looking out for rabbits, deer, fresh berries, wild greens, even cacti that could be cooked. These cowboy recipes were often wholesome and delicious. They were carried down through the generations into the modern ranch-wife's kitchen. She too had great pride in using only these natural ingredients along with her chicken's eggs and what ever she liked to grow in her garden.

This was the way it was for so very long. If you are of cowboy or ranch heritage, I am sure you remember your grandmothers basic cooking, maybe even your mother's, but what has happened in this last generation is an assault on our great heritage and definitely an assault on our health and our children's health.

So what happened? How did we get tricked into all this Non-food?

Well, that is, indeed, a good question! I think there are a few compound reasons but I am sure one of the biggest reasons started just after WWII. This was the time when the babies were booming and TV was just coming out. Mom and Grandma were amazed at how quiet and well behaved the children were as they watched their heroes like Roy Rogers, Gene Autrey, Hop-along Cassidy and The Lone Ranger ride to incredible victories.

This was good healthy stuff to watch on TV but the sponsors of these shows were anything but good and healthy for us. Remember "Twinkie the Kid"? (With a cowboy hat and rope) or how about the few million times you heard "Wonder Bread helps build strong bodies 12 ways"? Or what about the TV promotion that was just getting started with the catch phrase, "Better living through chemistry"?

One of the worst assaults that successfully targeted our youth is accredited to the soft drink, "Dr Pepper" (One of the highest sugar containing sodas) The "Good Doctor's" advice was on the label with a picture of a clock showing "10:00, 2:00 and 4:00" suggesting that you drink this around the clock at these times (3 bottles a day) every day to improve your health.

There were a ton of other sugar filled processed "cup cake delights" that had a shelf life of many years due to all the chemical preservatives. These were pushed along with new packaged snacks that had enough chemicals to "never go bad". And to top off all this, microwaveable instant meals were just coming in from left field.

Now with the kids being so well behaved while watching all this great wholesome stuff (Like Roy Rogers) on TV, Mom and even Grandma began to come to some of there own conclusions. As a child I remember overhearing my Grandma saying something to my mom like, *"Life seems to be going in a better direction lately. The kids are quiet and these new "modern miracle" instant foods, Wonder Bread, Hostess Twinkies, sugar coated cereals, and TV dinners must all be a part of this whole new "blessing from God" in this new modern age. These new foods must be good for you because modern science has "enriched" and "fortified" them with so many good vitamins! Before this, all our kids were ever getting from us was food made with plain old natural ingredients".*

Are you beginning to see where things went bad and how the media was responsible for tricking us into swallowing all these lies? All this stuff from the 50's and 60's led up to the sad predicament we now have.

You will notice that this chapter refers to "DANGEROUSLY processed foods." This is because, as I have stated, there ARE safe healthy ways to process good organic food. Safely canned organic foods and organic frozen vegetables can be great. Just be sure to read labels carefully. Look for that USDA Certified Organic logo.

However, mostly when we use the term "processed foods" in this book we will be referring to the 98.9% of processed foods which have been altered from their natural states in order to extend their shelf life. Many of these "foods" come in a box, can, bag, carton or jar and are processed to this condition mostly through chemicals. They are often very poor quality and usually cheap. About 90 percent of the money Americans spend on "food" is used to buy these edible, food-like substances.

I thank God that more and more of our supermarkets are making certified organic foods available. The Safeway Company has been very good about this and I have come to really appreciate many of the "Safeway Organics" products. (No I am not getting a "kick-back from Safeway!) The most important thing is that it has the USDA Certified Organic logo on it. If it does, all the dangerous forms of processing will have been eliminated. (Chemical additives, food from GMO crops or use of rancid oils etc) and you can safely know that you are eating real whole organic food.

Also I encourage all of you to get back to the basics of life as much as you can. Grow those gardens! You can do it. Make sure you grow them without pesticides and herbicides and that you use organic fertilizer only. Also learn how to safely "can" (with mason jars) and learn to freeze and store your harvests safely as well.

Cowboy up folks! We were all once like sheep led astray but if you have Jesus He will show you the way to live for Him. Many Christians forget that this INCLUDES keeping your bodies healthy and clean as Temples of The Holy Spirit! I have always wondered why Christians always seem to forget this part of God's instruction for us so easily.

But getting back to processed foods, one of the biggest problems is that many of these "edible food-like substances" will look just like good whole real food on the surface. This is until you start reading the labels (Which 95 percent of Americans never bother to do)

Even to the average shopper, many "meals in a box" are pretty obvious as being processed food but what about those jars that contain peanut butter or honey? What can they change in something basic like peanut butter or honey?

When peanut butter is real, the ingredients list will simply say, "Roasted Peanuts" which is all peanut butter ever needs. However finding it without hydrogenated oil and added sugar and sodium is almost impossible

CHAPTER 1: THE NEED FOR NUTRITION

You've heard the terms "hydrogenated" and "partially hydro-genated" used to describe oils. You've seen them on food labels and heard the warnings. Here's why you should avoid these chemically modified fats. You will find out that hundreds of doctors, researchers and scientists are blatantly warning us about the detrimental health effects of this ingredient. And you learn that this substance causes cancer, birth defects, heart disease, diabetes and many other fatal diseases.

Hydrogenation, complete or partial, is a chemical process in which hydrogen is added to liquid oils to turn them into a solid form. Partially hydrogenated fat molecules have trans-fats, and they are the worst type of fat you can consume. Don't confuse these man-made trans-fats with those that occur naturally in some foods. It is only these chemically altered trans-fats that are used in commercial peanut butter. (Such as "Jif" and "Skippy") For your health's sake please stay away from this stuff.

Real peanut butter is delicious and is a great source of protein. This author's breakfast almost always includes organic peanut butter and raw honey on whole organic Ezekiel bread. If I am really hungry my breakfast may include an egg or two from our own chickens who eat our organic food scraps. Ummmm- boy! Life could not be better!

I thank God for His bounty of healthy food. (And medicine) He has made all this available to us by his hand alone. All we have to do is simply eat only God's wonderful food and stay away from those "edible food-like substances" the media and government is pushing at us.

So what happens when we use dangerous chemical substances made from the process of distillation, isolation through centrifugal force, and other ways of changing the molecular structure? Well, put simply it becomes a "fake". Science likes to call this process "synthesis". They will also lie and tell you it is healthy.

All drugs on the market are now synthetic (Not made from a whole form of animal vegetable or mineral) and more and more of our food is becoming at least partly synthetic. Even if the main ingredients are natural enough, the ways of processing and preserving are almost always shown to be carcinogenic (containing a cancer causing substance)

Also, if the product lists any vitamins as *ingredients*, it means they are not found in the product naturally. So it now becomes a food product and not a real food. The vitamins used are always synthetically made and were added in an attempt to make the product look healthy. They were most likely added to cover up the fact that in the processing, the natural vitamins were completely destroyed. This is almost always the case in food products.

So for good nutrition, we must all simply learn to eat only real food and read the label to see if it is not. This does not seem to require a whole lot of sense, does it? If it has a list of ingredients (Other than animal vegetable or mineral) on the label, it is dangerously processed edible food-like substance and not real food. **If you can just begin to understand this you will add many more healthy happy years to your life.**

Processed foods have been altered from their natural state for reasons the FDA calls "safety" and for reasons the marketers call "convenience". And scary as it seems, about 90 percent of the money that Americans spend on food is used to buy these processed items. Have we just forgotten all about God's plan for our food and medicine on earth?

Food is great just the way it is made my God so why process it? Processed foods are more convenient and cheaper - that's what it comes down to. That is what suckers people in! It's seems so much easier to bake a cake by opening up a box, pouring out a dry mix, and adding an egg and some oil than starting from scratch.

Having Jambalaya in five minutes by pouring hot water into a carton can make cooking a breeze but convenience isn't the only thing you get when you eat processed foods like this. What you do get is very unhealthy and you get very unhealthy fast! Also your body starts to crave more of the very thing that is killing you. It becomes a deadly trap. Does this not sound like something Satan is involved in?

It is hard to start with what "foods" to quit eating but I will try to work off of what I have seen with my many good Christian cowboy and rancher friends. It is quite a list:

Packaged cookies, cakes and deserts: These are full of deadly trans-fats and hydrogenated oils which are used for long shelf-life. These seem to always be at the snack table at most cowboy churches and events. I am sorry folks, but this stuff is just real, real bad for you!

"Pringles" This is the all-time favorite "Cancer-in-a-Can" snack! Acrylamide, a cancer-causing and potentially neurotoxic chemical, is created when carbohydrate-rich foods (Such as potatoes) are cooked at high temperatures, whether baked, fried, roasted or toasted. Some of the worst offenders include potato chips and French fries, but many foods cooked or processed at temperatures above 212°F may contain acryl amide. Pringles are made from a mix of white rice, wheat, GMO corn and potato flakes and when they hit the high heat they are at the top of the list for creating this neurotoxin.

"Hamburger Helper" Organic grass fed beef is a wonderful healthy food and one of the best sources for protein we can have. As ranchers and cowboys many of us have a lot of access to this grade "A" food. I also believe that it is this beef that is helping to keep you healthy in spite of all the other stuff in many of your diets. However, I have actually seen people add "Hamburger Helper" to this wonderful food.

Read the label on hamburger helper products and you will see what these little "helpers" are really packed with MSG and many other chemicals.

But then again, MSG is in most all processed foods! The Campbell's soups, the Lays flavored potato chips, Top Ramen, Heinz canned gravy, Swanson frozen prepared meals, Kraft salad dressings, especially the 'healthy low fat' ones. The items that didn't have MSG had something called Hydrolyzed Vegetable Protein, which is just another name for Monosodium Glutamate. It was shocking to see just how many of the foods we feed our children everyday are filled with this stuff. They hide MSG under many different names in order to fool those who catch on.

People keep asking "What ingredients should I avoid?" So here is a list that covers a few of the most toxic and disease-promoting ingredients in the food supply.

These are the substances causing cancer, diabetes, heart disease and leading to tens of billions of dollars in unnecessary health care costs across America and around the world (Which, is very likely exactly why we find these in processed food)

Acrylamides: Toxic, cancer-causing chemicals formed in foods when carbohydrates are exposed to high heat (baking, frying, grilling). They're present in everything from bread crusts to snack chips, and because they aren't intentional ingredients, acrylamides do NOT have to be listed on labels.

Autolyzed Proteins: Highly processed form of protein containing free glutamate and used to mimic the taste-enhancer chemical MSG.

Benzene: This is a well known cancer-causing chemical and studies have shown it to be responsible for hundreds of thousands of deaths from leukemia and other cancers. This is formed when Sodium benzoate (used in many processed foods as a preservative) and ascorbic acid. (Disguised as natural vitamin C) are combined. This occurs in many citrus flavored drinks and sodas and is most prominent in powdered drinks like Country Time Lemonade.

BPA (Bisphenol-A): A hormone mimicking chemical found in nearly all food packaging plastics. Active in just parts per billion, BPA promotes cancer, infertility and hormone disorders. It also "feminizes" males, promoting male breast growth and hormone disruption.

Casein: Milk proteins. Hilariously, this is widely used in "soy cheese" products that claim to be alternatives to cow's milk. Nearly all of them are made with cow's milk proteins.

Corn Syrup: Just another name for High Fructose Corn Syrup (see below). This is frequently used in infant formula products.

Food Colors: FD&C Red #40, for example, is linked to behavioral disorders in children. Nearly all artificial food colors are derived from petroleum, and many are contaminated with aluminum.

Genetically Modified Ingredients: Not currently listed on the label because the GMO industry (Monsanto and DuPont) absolutely does not want people to know which foods contain GMOs. Nearly all conventionally grown corn, soy and cotton are now GMOs. They're linked to severe infertility problems and may even cause the bacteria in your body to produce and release a pesticide in your own gut. **If you're not eating organic labeled corn, you're definitely eating GMO corn. Stay alive and eat only certified organic corn.**

High Fructose Corn Syrup: A highly processed liquid sugar extracted with the chemical solvent glutaraldehyde and frequently contaminated with mercury. It's also linked to diabetes, obesity and mood disorders. Used in thousands of grocery items, including things you wouldn't suspect like pizza sauce and salad dressings.

Hydrochloride: When you see anything hydrochloride, such as Pyridoxine Hydrochloride or Thiamin Hydrochloride, those are chemical forms of B vitamins that companies add to their products to be able to claim higher RDA values of vitamins. But these are synthetic, chemical forms of vitamins, not real vitamins from foods or plants. Nutritionally, they are near-useless and may actually be bad for you. Also watch out for niacinamide and cyanocobalamin (synthetic vitamin B-12).

Hydrolyzed Vegetable Protein: This is a highly processed form of (usually) soy protein (Almost all soy is now GMO) that's processed to bring out the free glutamate (MSG). Used as a taste enhancer.

Partially Hydrogenated Oils: Oils that are modified using a chemical catalyst to make them stable at room temperature. This creates trans-fatty acids and greatly increases the risk of blocked arteries. It also promotes what we call "sludge blood," which is thick, viscous blood that's hard to pump. This is usually diagnosed by doctors as "high blood pressure" and (stupidly) treated with blood-thinning medications that are technically the same chemicals as rat poison (warfarin).

Phosphoric Acid: The acid used in sodas to dissolve the carbon dioxide and add to the overall fizzy-ness of the soda. Phosphoric acid will eat steel nails. It's also used by stone masons to etch rocks. The military uses it to clean the rust off battleships. In absolutely destroys tooth enamel. Search Google Images for "Mountain Dew Mouth" to see photos of teeth rotted out by phosphoric acid.

Propylene Glycol: A liquid used in the automotive industry to winterize RVs. It's also used to make the fake blueberries you see in blueberry muffins, bagels and breads. (Combined with artificial colors and corn syrup)

Sodium (Salt): The processed white salt lacking in trace minerals. In the holistic nutrition industry, we call it "death salt" because it promotes disease and death. Real salt, on the other hand, such as "dirty" sea salt or pink Himalayan salt, is loaded with the trace minerals that prevent disease, such as selenium (cancer), chromium (diabetes) and zinc (infectious disease). Much like with bread and sugar, white salt is terrible for your health. And don't be fooled by claims of "sea salt" in grocery stores. All salt came from the sea if you go far back enough in geologic time, so they can slap the "sea salt" claim on ANY salt!

Sodium Nitrite: A cancer-causing red coloring chemical added to bacon, hot dogs, sausage, beef jerky, ham, lunch meats, pepperoni and nearly all processed meats. Strongly linked to brain tumors, pancreatic cancers and colon cancers, the USDA once tried to ban it from the food supply but was out-maneuvered by the meat industry, which now dominates USDA regulations. Sodium nitrite is a complete poison used to make meats look fresh. Countless children die of cancer each year from sodium nitrite-induced cancers.

Soy Protein: Most all soy is now GMO. This is the number 1 protein source used in "protein bars," including many bars widely consumed by bodybuilders. This is so far away from health food that it is scary. Soy protein is the "junk protein" of the food industry. It's made from genetically modified (GMO) soybeans and then subjected to hexane, a chemical solvent that can literally explode.

Sucralose: An artificial chemical sweetener sold as Splenda. The sucralose molecule contains a chlorine atom. Researchers have repeatedly found that artificial sweeteners make people fat by actually promoting weight gain.

Sugar: I am not talking about raw sugar made from organic cane juice which is really just fine for us in moderation. I'm talking about the bleached, nutritionally-deficient byproduct of cane processing. During sugar cane processing, nearly all the minerals and vitamins end up in the blackstrap molasses that's usually fed to farm animals. (Blackstrap molasses is actually the "good" part of sugar cane juice.)

Molasses is often fed to farm animals because every cowboy and rancher knows that farm animals need good nutrition to stay alive. Amazingly, conventional doctors don't yet realize this about humans (Or they are ignoring it for some reason) and they continue to claim that eating white processed sugar is perfectly fine for you. This sugar promotes diabetes, obesity, mood disorders and nutritional deficiencies.

Textured Vegetable Protein: Usually made of soy protein which is extracted from genetically modified soybeans and then processed using hexane, an explosive chemical solvent (see soy protein, above). Widely used in vegetarian foods such as "veggie burgers" (most of which also contain MSG or yeast extract, by the way).

Yeast Extract: A hidden form of MSG that contains free glutamate and is used in many "natural" food products to claim "No MSG!" Yeast extract contains up to 14% free glutamate. You'll find it in thousands of grocery store products, from soups to snack chips.

Unbelievable! Aborted human cells are now used in the production of many common beverages;

The Obama Administration has given its blessing to Pepsi Co to continue utilizing the services of a company that produces flavor chemicals for the beverage giant using aborted human fetal tissue.

The following is from Mike Adams of Natural News:

LifeSiteNews.com reports that the Obama Security and Exchange Commission (SEC) has decided that PepsiCo's arrangement with San Diego, Cal.-based Senomyx, which produces flavor enhancing chemicals for Pepsi using human embryonic kidney tissue, simply constitutes "or-dinary business operations."

The issue began in 2011 when the non-profit group Children of God for Life (CGL) first broke the news about Pepsi's alliance with Senomyx, which led to massive outcry and a worldwide boycott of Pepsi products. At that time, it was revealed that Pepsi had many other options at its disposal to produce flavor chemicals, which is what its competitors do, but had instead chosen to continue using aborted fetal cells — or as Senomyx deceptively puts it, "isolated human taste receptors"

A few months later, Pepsi' shareholders filed a resolution pe-titioning the company to "adopt a corporate policy that recognizes human rights and employs ethical standards which do not involve using the remains of aborted human beings in both private and col-laborative research and development agreements." But the Obama Administration shut down this 36-page proposal, deciding instead that Pepsi's used of aborted babies to flavor its beverage products is just business as usual, and not a significant concern.

"We're not talking about what kind of pencils PepsiCo wants to use — we are talking about exploiting the remains of an aborted child for profit," said Debi Vinnedge, Executive Director of CGL, concern-ing the SEC decision. "Using human embryonic kidney (HEK-293) to produce flavor enhancers for their beverages is a far cry from routine operations!"

To be clear, the aborted fetal tissue used to make Pepsi's flavor chemicals does not end up in the final product sold to customers, according to reports — it is used, instead, to evaluate how actual human taste receptors respond to these chemical flavorings. But the fact that Pepsi uses them at all when viable, non-human alternatives are available illustrates the company's blatant disregard for ethical and moral concerns in the matter.

Back in January, Oklahoma Senator Ralph Shortey proposed legislation to ban the production of aborted fetal cell-derived flavor chemicals in his home state. If passed, S.B. 1418 would also reportedly ban the sale of any products that contain flavor chemicals derived from human fetal tissue, which includes Pepsi products as well as products produced by Kraft and Nestle. End Natural News

Let's Take a Closer Look at Country Time "Lemonade"

A good example of one of the most highly dangerous of processed food products is Country Time Lemonade by Kraft Foods. This is at the very top of the list for dangerous food products containing the known cancer causing substance, benzene.

Sodium benzoate is used in many processed foods as a preservative and is very prominent in *Country Time Lemonade*. However, this product also contains a lot of ascorbic acid. (Disguised as natural vitamin C) These two chemicals actually **form** the chemical known as benzene when combined together. **Benzene is a well known cancer-causing chemical and studies have shown it to be responsible for hundreds of thousands of deaths from leukemia and other cancers.**

The FDA knew of the problem as early as 1990, but never made the findings public. Instead, the FDA came to an agreement with the US soft drinks association that the soft drink industry would reformulate the drinks. In recent months, private tests have been done, and support claims by a former chemist for Cadbury

Schweppes, who, as Beverage Daily reports, is now saying they will blow the whistle on the benzene levels in soft drinks and the health risks involved. (So far it has not happened)

Many other soft drinks with lots of ascorbic acid in them are just as dangerous due to that fact that they almost all use Sodium benzoate as a preservative.

The FDA now admits: "Benzene, which is used to make glues, paints and detergents, has been linked to leukemia and other cancers of the blood" How nice of them to now admit it when God knows how many people have died from the many soft drinks carrying this deadly poison. **Please start reading labels and understanding them; it could save you and your family's life!**

The healthy alternative is real lemonade! It is not much trouble at all to make and it is really quite easy. (and fun) Just squeeze a few lemons into water and add a small amount of real organic raw cane sugar. Take a little time and save a lot of your time on earth!

If you can't afford a lot of lemons remember that only a few lemons in a gallon or two of water will still taste quite strong. It is kind of like "fishes and loaves". If you really don't have the time to make it there are many good organic real lemonades available in bottles for just a little more money. One of the best tasting and healthy real lemonades I have found is *Safeway Organics* brand. This is one great value for both taste and health!

Real Lemons are Good Medicine!

In sharp contrast to Country Time Lemonade, did you know that drinking a lot of real lemon juice (Yes, even in the form of true fresh lemonade) can actually dissolve gallstones and kidney stones over a few weeks time? Isn't this better than doing the FDA's dirty work of spreading cancer causing chemicals into the bodies of your Christian friends?

Accumulated toxins in the liver, gallbladder, kidneys, and other parts of the body can be flushed out using lemons, they are considered to be ideal for detoxification of the body.

Also, the juice of lemons is excellent and effective remedy to treat disorders of the throat and persistent catarrh. It is possible to prevent common colds at the first sign of a cold, if the affected person drinks a glass (or two or three) of warm and sugarless lemonade from the juice of one whole lemon.

Lemons are excellent for the treatment of cases of Putrefaction, particularly when it concerns disorders in the liver. Lemons in many cases really help in stirring up any of the latent toxins accumulated inside the body which cannot be eliminated by any other means. Consuming lemon juice is of great value when it is necessary to be rid of the impurities and the fermentative effects of an impaired liver.

The lemon is considered to be one of the most alkalinizing foods known, even though it has so much acid. Important nutrients such as potassium and vitamin B1 are also found in high amounts in the lemon. Citric acid also makes up about five to six per cent of the juice and tissues of lemons and limes; this percentage is very high compared to oranges at about one to one and a half percent, or the grapefruit, at about one to two percent citric acid.

Resistance in the body and the immune system are also boosted by consumption of lemons, it also aids in digestion and buffers the body against toxins .All types of fevers can be effectively cured using the lemon as a remedy. The citric acid present in the lemon engages and strengthens the feverish body better than any other nutrient. The elimination of toxins via the skin is increased by the lemon, this helps in reducing the fever affecting a person. The lemon juice is also an effective germicide and induces certain effects on the infective germ life brought on by influenza. The use of lemon juice alone is in fact, capable of defeating at many different types of infective germs in the human body.

A case for lemons and getting rid of gallstones:

My wife and I have a friend that had a very painful right side. She went to a doctor and was diagnosed with many gallstones. They wanted to do surgery and remove the gallbladder as they had done to her sister.

Being an herbalist, I tried to give her a strong tincture of the herb known as "Golden Coin Grass" (Jin Can Cao) which can be very effective in dissolving gallstones. I am sure it would have worked for her but she was poor financially and although we tried to give it to her for free she would not accept it. She worked at a Safeway store and asked if there was anything she could do that did not cost much money. My wife immediately said lemons, drink as much fresh juice as you can handle for a month or more.

She had a good connection to lemons working in the produce department so she took it to heart! She squeezed the juice of 3-4 lemons in water and put it in a one of those large "sip-cups" with a straw and walked around working and sipping on that all day, every day! (She may have gone through as many as 6 lemons a day) She said after a few days the pain went away. After about 6 weeks of this she went back to the doc and they could not find a trace of gallstones!

Please note: The popular "lemon juice/olive oil flush" that takes a few days is probably a good cleanse but even people that have been diagnosed with "no gallstones at all" get those little green balls showing up. This is not "Gallstones" but most likely just congealed food-stuff from the combo of lemon juice and olive oil.

Although Country Time Lemonade may be at the top of the list as a dangerous packaged food item, there is a type of home processing that is done in so many homes today that it may truly be the number one cause of bad general health in America. We are talking about simply eating or drinking water or liquids that have been warmed in a microwave oven.

Microwave Oven Cooked Food ; The Deadly Curse of Convenience

As an active member of a cowboy church I am at a lot of horse events and other gatherings. When walking around, I can't help but notice all the horse trailer rigs and RVs with a generator and the perfect little shelf-space with a microwave oven in it. I have also seen these ovens in a lot of bunk-houses and sadly even in the kitchens of most ranch wife's homes and even pastor's homes.

I mention this first because I am very familiar with cowboys and most of us would rather avoid reading this whole chapter than give up that perfect microwave shelf-space for warming up a meal on those cold mornings before a round-up or event.

Well, in many ways, I don't blame you. What you are about to read may be so shocking that you will never use a microwave oven again in your life. However there is good news! You don't have to give up that shelf-space for fast cooking when you need it!

The new convection/toaster ovens are exactly the same size so they fit right in the same space, use just about the same amount of electricity and are now almost as fast at warming or cooking something as a microwave. And the price is no more (Even a bit less) than a microwave to replace. We have an RV and we replaced the microwave with a nifty convection/toaster oven for around $69.00. It works great, fit in the space great and it is perfectly safe to eat food that has been warmed or cooked in it.

In a recent survey, when asked what was most important in deciding "what to do for dinner" such as price, taste, nutrition, or convenience, an overwhelming 70% said convenience. The survey did not say but I suspect to most people that means "popped in the microwave" or a trip through a drive-through fast food place.

Now surely popping something in the microwave at home couldn't hurt you even if there was no nutrition left in it, right? Wouldn't they warn us or ban microwave ovens if eating food cooked in them was a major health threat? Well, the data may shock you but here are the facts:

This data I discovered has confirmed just about all my suspicions. I believe that at least in part, the general obesity in this country, the lack of energy, and highly increased cancers of all kinds along with all the new "designer diseases" can be traced to our habit of eating food and water warmed in microwave ovens.

In a paper called "Comparative Study of Food Prepared Conventionally and in the Microwave Oven" published by Raum & Zelt in1992, it states: "PRODUCTION OF UNNATURAL MOLECULES IS INEVITABLE" Naturally occurring amino acids have been observed to undergo isomeric changes (changes in shape - morphing) as well as transformation into toxic forms, under the impact of microwaves produced in ovens. This is like eating something totally different than our God created for us.

One short-term study found significant and disturbing changes in the blood of individuals consuming microwaved milk and vegetables. Eight volunteers ate various combinations of the same foods cooked different ways. All foods that were processed through the microwave ovens caused changes in the blood of the volunteers. Hemoglobin levels decreased and overall white cell levels and cholesterol levels increased. Lymphocytes decreased. Luminescent (light-emitting) bacteria were employed to detect energetic changes in the blood. Significant increases were found in the luminescence of these bacteria when exposed to blood serum obtained after the consumption of microwaved food."

The following is a summary of the Russian investigations on microwave ovens:

Carcinogens were formed in virtually all foods tested. No test food was subjected to more microwaving than necessary to accomplish the purpose, i.e., cooking, thawing, or heating to ensure sanitary ingestion.

Here's a summary of some of the results:

- Microwaving prepared meats sufficiently to ensure sanitary ingestion caused formation of d-Nitrosodiethanolamines, a well-known carcinogen.
- Microwaving milk and cereal grains converted some of their amino acids into carcinogens.
- Thawing frozen fruits converted their glucoside and galactoside containing fractions into carcinogenic substances.
- Extremely short exposure of raw, cooked or frozen vegetables converted their plant alkaloids into carcinogens.
- Carcinogenic free radicals were formed in microwaved plants, especially root vegetables.

So who invented the microwave oven? It turns out it was the Nazis who actually invented these ovens. (Why am I not surprised?) They were used in their mobile support calling them the "radiomissor". These ovens were to be used for the invasion of Russia. By using electronic equipment for preparation of meals on a mass scale, the logistical problem of cooking fuels would have been eliminated, as well as the convenience of producing edible products in a greatly reduced time-factor.

After the war, Dr. Percy Spencer, a self-taught engineer with the Raytheon Corporation, claimed to have "invented" the microwave oven in 1946. The Raytheon Corporation did actually file the first U.S. patent on one. The first ones were called "Radar Ranges" in 1954.

How Microwave Ovens Work:

All microwave ovens contain a magnetron which is a tube in which electrons are affected by magnetic and electric fields. They produce micro wavelength radiation at about 2450 Megahertz (MHz) or 2.45 Gigahertz (GHz). This microwave radiation interacts with the molecules in food. The wave energy inside the oven changes polarity from positive to negative with each cycle of the wave. These changes of polarity happen millions of times every second. Food molecules (especially the molecules of water) have a positive and negative end just like a magnet has a north and a south polarity.

As these microwaves generated from the magnetron "bombard" the food at nearly the speed of light, they cause the polar molecules in the food or water to rotate at the same frequency millions of times a second.

This is major agitation! For example, much less agitation is used in pharmaceutical drug labs to separate or isolate molecules in the making of just about any thing they want. This agitation creates the molecular friction, which heats up the food. The friction also causes substantial damage to the surrounding molecules, often tearing them apart or forcefully deforming them. The scientific name for this deformation is "structural isomerism". If you think that water warmed in a microwave is safe please think again. It is water molecules (H-2-o) that are the most dangerously altered.

It makes absolutely no sense to me that our FDA is "looking out for us" and yet has not even mentioned the dangers of the worst cancer producing machines in history.

Some of you may say, "OK so what can I do? I don't have time to cook on a real stove" Please try to understand that **all you have on this earth is time.** And you will add years to your time on earth by preparing your food from WHOLE FOOD scratch and on a real stove.

Also remember that cooking can be a lot of fun! I have not come to that knowledge myself because my wife absolutely loves to cook and if I try to help she chases me out of the kitchen.

If you really need to cook something or warm something that fast (And there are times we do) please just replace it with one of those new convection/toaster ovens available at very little cost. Just get one and take your microwave down to your backyard shooting range. Now that is a fun and healthy experience you can have with your microwave!

Getting back to wholesome food and good nutrition:

With all the fake processed "food" it is sometimes hard to grasp a reality of what real food is. The bible is always a good place to go for a reality check. So before we get into cooking let's take a quick look at all the food mentioned in the bible. I am pretty sure you won't find canned biscuits and Pringles.

- Almonds---Genesis 43:11; Numbers 17:8
- Anise---Matthew 23:23
- Apples---Song of Solomon 2:5; Joel 1:12
- Barley---Ruth 2:23
- Barley Bread---2 Kings 4:42

- Beans or Pulse, also known as Legumes---2 Samuel 17:28;
- Beef---Deuteronomy 14:4
- Bitter Herbs (dandelion greens, watercress, arugula, parsley, cilantro)---Exodus 12:8
- Bison (Pygarg)---Deuteronomy 14:5
- Bread---Luke 22:19
- Butter---Isaiah 7:22
- Carob (St. John's Bread)---Matthew3:4; Mark 1:6 (akris: this Greek word for locusts can apply to either an insect or the top of a tree or plant. Many believe this to be St. John's Bread or Carob which grew wild around the river Jordan. It is named for John the Baptist).
- Cinnamon---Exodus 30:23
- Coriander---Exodus 16:31; Numbers 11:7
- Corn---Ruth 2:14; I Samuel 17:17
- Cheese---I Samuel 17:18
- Chicken---Matthew 23:37
- Cinnamon---Exodus 30:23; Revelations 18:13
- Cucumbers---Numbers 11:5
- Cumin or Cummin---Isaiah 28:25
- Curds (Cottage and Ricotta Cheese)---Genesis 18:8
- Dates---2 Samuel 6:19
- Dill---Matthew 23:23
- Dried Fruits---Genesis 3:2
- Eggs---Job 6:6
- Figs---Numbers 13:23; I Samuel 25:18
- Fish with Scales (Anchovies, Bass, Cod, Flounder, Haddock, Halibut, Herring, Mackerel, Orange Roughy,

Perch, Pike, Pollack, Salmon, Sardines, Tilapia, Trout, Tuna, Turbot, Whitefish & Whiting, among others)---Deuteronomy 14:9; Leviticus 11:9

- Flax Seed---Exodus 9:31
- Flour (Whole Meal)---Ezekiel 16:19; Numbers 6:15
- Fruits (All)---Genesis 1:29
- Garlic---Numbers 11:5
- Goat---Deuteronomy 14:4
- Grapes---Deuteronomy 24:21
- Grape Juice (New Wine)---Zechariah 9:17
- Grasshoppers, Crickets & Locusts---Leviticus 11:22
- Herbs (Leafy Plants) and Vegetables---Genesis 1:29; Proverbs 15:17
- Herbs (Used as Medicine) EZ. 47:12 the original word used in EZ. 47:12 is t-e-r-v-w-p-h-ah, and it means: a remedy. The original Hebrew word used for medicine in Proverbs 17:22 is listed as word #1456 in Strong's concordance. The Hebrew spelling is g-e-h-a-h and it means: a cure. Ps.104:14 says that he has given us "herbs for the service of Man"
- Herbs (Seasonings)---Proverbs 27:25; Matthew 13:32
- Honey---Proverbs 24:13; Proverbs 25:16 (warning to use moderation)
- Hyssop (Capers)---Psalms 51:7; John 19:29
- Lamb & Sheep---Deuteronomy 14:4
- Leeks---Numbers 11:5
- Lentils---Genesis 25:34
- Leaven (Yeast)---Leviticus 23:17; Galatians 5:9

- Marjoram(Hyssop)---Exodus 12:22
- Meats---Deuteronomy 14; Leviticus 11
- Melon---Numbers 11:5
- Milk---Isaiah 7:21-22
- Millet---Ezekiel 4:9
- Mint---Matthew 23:23; Luke 11:42
- Mulberry---2 Samuel 5:24; 1 Chorinthians 14:14
- Mustard Seeds---Mark 4:31; Luke 13:19
- Nuts---Song of Solomon 6:11
- Olives and Olive Oil---Leviticus 2:4; Deuteronomy 8:8
- Onions---Numbers 11:5
- Pistachio Nuts---Genesis 43:11
- Pomegranates---Numbers 13:23
- Poultry including Chicken, Duck, Goose, Pheasant, Pigeons, Quail, Turkey---Deuteronomy 14:11
- Quail---Exodus 16:13
- Raisins---2 Samuel 16:1
- Rye---Isaiah 28:25
- Saffron---Song of Solomon 4:14
- Salt---Leviticus 2:13; Luke 14:34
- Sourdough Bread---Leviticus 23:17; Amos 4:5
- Spelt (Fitches)---Ezekiel 4:9
- Spices---1 Kings 10:10
- Squash (Gourds)---2 Kings 4:39
- Sweet Cane (Sucanat or Evaporated Cane Juice)---Isaiah 43:24; Jeremiah 6:20
- Unleavened Bread (Tortillas, Flat Bread, Chapatis)---Genesis, 19:3; Exodus 29:2

- Venison---Deuteronomy 14:5
- Vinegar---Ruth 2:14
- Water---Genesis 21:19; John 4:7
- Wheat---Ruth 2:23; Psalm 81:16
- Wheat bread---Exodus 29:2
- Wine---John 2:1-10, 1 Timothy 5:23
- Yogurt (butter of Kine)---Deuteronomy 32:14

The Forbidden Food in The Old Testament :

- Blood---Leviticus 7:26
- Camel---Leviticus 11:4
- Catfish---Deuteronomy 14:10
- Fat from animals---Leviticus 7:23
- Fish without Scales---Leviticus 11:12
- Ostrich & Emu---Leviticus 11:13
- Pork or Swine---Leviticus 11:7
- Rabbit---Leviticus 11:6
- Shellfish (shrimp, crab, lobster, clams etc. . .)---Leviticus 11:12
- Snail---Leviticus 11:30
- Tortoise---Leviticus 11:29

So what is a good example of eating nutritionally right?

Well, if I can't use my own life as an example I guess I shouldn't be writing this book! So it is my pleasure to tell you how and why my wife and I feel so great and how my wonderful wife Heidi, (Who fortunately loves to cook) keeps us feeling this way.

It is through her keen and natural awareness of true wholesome food and nutrition. It is not a scientifically laid out plan, (Neither one of us is good at that sort of thing) it is more like just having a feel for what is right and what is wrong as applied to the temple of the Holy Spirit which is our bodies.

And no, we are certainly not perfect on this but the fact that we are not perfect is a key to why it is so important to just TRY to stay healthy from good common sense and a little bit of knowledge. (In fact the "knowledge" I am talking about is really just "un-learning" what the media and life in the "NORM" has crammed into your brain)

Of course one of the concerns to many people is the cost of an all organic diet. Well I will be the first to tell you we are not 100% organic but maybe about 80 - 90%. It breaks down about like this: 95% of our dairy products, 100% of any canned food, (canned food is very important to be organic) about 90% of our meat. (Which we tend to eat a lot of) No vegetarians here! 100% of all our produce (Much of which is from our own garden) 90% of our grains and 60 % of our nuts, 100% of our mustard and ketchup, 100% of our salad dressings, 100% of our cooking oils (Exclusively extra virgin olive oil, coconut oil and grape seed oil). Grape seed oil is one of the only oils that will never produce trans-fats at even the highest cooking temperature. By the way, **ALL** canola oil is now GMO which is why it is never considered in our house. Also, we do not eat a lot of sugar but we are not afraid of it. We use 100% organic sugar made from cane juice. (Keeping it in moderation of course)

With all of this considered we closely figured that it is costing us maybe as much as 20% more than if we did not use mostly organic food. This is totally amazing to me because I would not trade this health for any amount of money! We never get sick and we can work long hours and do not get tired. If you are a bit on the low income side please find something you can give up to make up for that 20%. Trust me, it is worth it!

Besides just the organic food factor we eat a large amount of fresh garlic and a large amount of olive oil almost daily. It is incorporated into many of our delicious meals or at least in our daily salads. I think one reason we are both blessed with great health is the fact that my wife uses only fresh crushed garlic and she uses it in just about everything she makes! (OK, maybe not ice cream) She always uses that garlic press on fresh cloves of garlic! Nothing else such as garlic powder would ever even be considered! Fresh garlic is natural medicine that not only keeps you from getting sick but it is tonic to your body.

I believe that using fresh garlic in this way is a very big key to health! So many great healthy meals can be simply made from organic whole grain pasta with fresh garlic, olive oil and REAL BUTTER. This is great by itself or you can throw in almost any sautéed organic vegetable or meat, sprinkle a little organic cheese and have an endless source of easily prepared meals that are extremely nutritious and absolutely delicious. One of the biggest keys to making the organic change is to become **nutritionally creative!** This will make it fun and you will discover everything tastes so much better now that you can make it your way.

By the way, another big key to health is always using REAL BUTTER (Organic of course) instead of margarine. Ounce you read the process below of how they make the "alternative" known as margarine you will never want to even LOOK at margarine again.

The Triple Toxic Poisonous Process of Making Margarine

Today, the production of margarine is an unappetizing process which uses several toxic chemicals. Here's an overview of the steps involved:

Vegetable oil is made from oil seeds such as soybeans, corn, cottonseed or canola. (All of which are now GMO)

The seeds are cleaned and crushed and the oil is extracted by applying high temperatures and pressure.

Since heat and light accelerate the rate of the reaction between polyunsaturated oils and oxygen, this extraction process causes the oils to become rancid, producing unpleasant and noxious odors and flavors.

Any oil left in the seed pulp is removed with dangerous solvents such as hexane, a known neurotoxin.

The crude oil is then de-gummed with acid to remove other impurities, and a caustic soda is added to remove the de-gumming acids.

The resulting gray and smelly oil is bleached with Fuller's earth (the same ingredient used in cat litter) and then filtered.

The rancid smells are removed through a high temperature steam cleaning deodorization process. This destroys any remaining nutrients and antioxidants.

The refined oil is mixed with a nickel catalyst and subjected to hydrogen gas in a high pressure, high temperature reactor.

The high temperature and pressure in the presence of the nickel catalyst forces hydrogen atoms into the oil molecules, creating a partially solid, saturated product. This process is called hydrogenation. It is at this point that super dangerous trans-fats are created. Basically, the artificially created saturated fat molecules always bond in the wrong places within our bodies causing everything from cancer to heart attacks to brain strokes. These molecular misfits have been linked to inflammation, blood platelet stickiness, insulin resistance and many other life threatening health problems.

The resulting gray, smelly grease is filtered to remove the leftover toxic nickel and other suspended materials. The grease is then mixed with soap-like emulsifiers, then steam cleaned to remove the obnoxious odors.

The mixture is then bleached to remove the gray color, and artificial flavors, synthetic vitamins and colors are added to improve the appearance and taste. The mixture is now extruded into plastic tubs for sale.

Finally, clever advertising and marketing campaigns are implemented to promote the final product as a "health food" to the unsuspecting public, usually with the full endorsement of many scientists, doctors, nutritionists and health authorities. These are what I like to call "NEWTS" (New Experts With Ties) Why do they always wear ties?

As you can see from the process above, these toxic spreads are NOT health foods, and should be avoided like the plague! Instead, just use real, clean organic butter, preferably in raw or cultured form. Besides, butter tastes so darn good. Thank you Lord!

What about those artificial sweeteners?

The laws governing the sale of drugs and food additives in the USA require all substances be safe for human consumption. This may actually be one of the few laws that at least seem to make sense as far as making sure that we aren't mass-poisoned by some wacked-out food product company. It is a simple decent law to protect our citizens, isn't it? So, certainly artificial sweeteners like "NutraSweet" (aspartame) and others should pose no danger to us at all, right?

Well the truth is the artificial sweetener aspartame primarily consumed in soda and other beverages and as a popular sugar substitute has CONSISENTLY been found to cause tumors and brain seizures in animal subject tests.

In 2005, a European Cancer Research Center, the Ramazzini Foundation, called for an urgent re-examination of aspartame in food and beverages to protect children. This call is made in the face of the US FDA's stand that aspartame is safe for human consumption on the ground that "aspartame as a carcinogen is not supported by data."

Yet as early as 1960, in our own country, aspartame has been found to create holes in brain tissue, adversely affect the brain and nerve development in the fetus, cause cancer, migraines, headaches, seizures, convulsions and even retinal damage. With this amount of negative findings, aspartame should have been removed from the market years ago!

The facts are, few people know that in 1960 aspartame was indeed removed from the market after it was already approved for limited use based on tests selected by Searle, the company who originally produced the artificial sweetener. This was after Dr. John Olney, a research psychiatrist from Washington School of Medicine, revealed that consumption of aspartic acid (the major ingredient in aspartame) produced holes in the brains of animal subjects.

In April 1981, Dr. Arthur Hayes was appointed the new Commissioner for the FDA and he later approved aspartame for use in dry goods. In 1983, he also approved aspartame for use in diet drinks, conveniently leaving months later to work for Searle's advertising agency.

In 1985 none other than the notorious Monsanto Company purchased G. D. Searle and Company. It then became the NutraSweet Company who was the manufacturer of Aspartame. This notorious neuro-toxin sold to the public as an artificial sweetener had fallen into the hands of perhaps one of the most evil organizations in the world.

Monsanto is also responsible for all the genetically modified foods that are at the brink of poisoning most of the crops on earth. You will come to understand a lot about Monsanto in the next few chapters so be prepared to deal with one of those organizations of this world that is very dark and a bit scary.

The Benefits of Eating Only Organic Non-GMO foods

Without all the nutritionally worthless fast food and processed food that is advertised there would not be much of a media left when you think about it. This is because media has thrived on the money for commercials from the multitude of worthless processed food items. All these products rely on cheap fast grown bulk food that relies on deadly chemicals to make it all happen.

The main aspect that most people are concerned about is simply whether the food in question was grown with pesticides, herbicides, or chemical fertilizers and whether that food contains pesticide/herbicide residues on the actual food when you eat it. This is, of course, a very important concern.

The evidence is now stacked way over the media's heads and it is no longer a question scientifically. It is now a proven fact that any and all food grown with these chemicals contains residue when it is eaten. What IS a real question is, how long will the FDA, the media, and the food giants keep up their "smile of denial" and continue lying to us?

The disastrous health consequences are also proven to be both potentially carcinogenic (cancer causing) and containing corrupt sex hormones that can cause one to become sterile. They can cause unusually fast development in females (With girls getting their periods at 8 years old and growing breasts) They can also cause male-like features in women and female like features in men.

Another MAJOR aspect of organic vs. conventional food is the impacts of conventional farm chemicals on our American soil. (This can ruin the soil for generations to come)

The harsh chemical fertilizers, pesticides, and herbicides used in conventional farming can destroy a large part of the microbial activity in the soils (bacteria and fungi) that help to make soil minerals more available to the plants roots. Modern conventional farming degrades this aspect of the soil which results in very low micro-nutrient levels in the vegetables that you eat. This will result in "empty food" that makes your body weaker and weaker as it is fooled into thinking it is getting nutrition.

With organic farming, these harsh chemicals are never used, and the soil is healthy and biologically active (fungi and bacteria aid the plant roots with much more uptake of minerals and nutrients), and the plant's roots can therefore obtain real nutrition. This produces foods with much higher micro-nutrient levels.

Also, the heavy uses of chemical fertilizers cause crops to grow much faster than normal, leading to a shallow root system. This shallow root system can not absorb much of anything. (even if it there is anything in the burnt out soil to absorb)

This is compared to organically raised crops that have deep extensive root systems to obtain all of the nutrients the plant needs. And here is the real kicker: Organic food is really nothing more than food grown the way God intended it to grow. Nothing is added, it is just absent of cancer causing, sexual altering, deadly chemicals that should only be thought up in science fiction movies!

Are you beginning to get the picture? Is it worth a little extra cost? WELL DUH! (Please excuse the over-literate expletive)

But sadly this is not even half of the story. What they have now done to our nation's seeds are like the scariest sci-fi movie you could imagine but unfortunately it is not fiction at all. This next chapter was a very sad wakeup call even for me. As I did the research I was almost in a state of shock!

It is hard to believe that this country which I dearly love is the only country in the world so vigorously promoting the end to all wholesome and healthy natural food crops as we know them. I sincerely hope the upcoming chapters will make a difference in many of your lives and help keep many of you healthy and happy for many years to come.

CHAPTER 2:
THE SATANIC ATTACK ON
OUR FOOD SUPPLY

Our Expanding Genetically Modified (GMO) food supply

So what are GMO's? Genetically modified organisms, or GMOs, are created when a gene from one species is transferred to another, creating something that would not be found in nature.

A large percentage of domestic crops (up to 95% of soybean and corn yields) have DNA that was tweaked in a lab, yet it is nearly impossible to know which food items contain these genetically engineered ingredients. Many are even genetically engineered to contain herbicides like roundup in their actual DNA structure.

It is beyond me why food items that contain GMOs are not even labeled in America. Why so sneaky? The European Union has banned GMOs, as have Australia, Japan, the UK and dozens of other countries that recognize the disastrous health defects associated with GMO and actually care about their citizens.

In fact it is America and our wonderful FDA that is leading the way to world destruction from this deadly idea of GMO crops. WHY AMERICA? This totally breaks my heart and I can only look to our almighty God for answers.

So how do we prevent eating these potentially deadly GMO foods if they are unlabeled? Your best defense is to purchase (or grow) certified organic food, which cannot, by law, contain any GMOs in order to be certified. And you need to tell your friends and loved ones to do the same. It only costs a little more but it is more than worth it. If you grow your food or your cattle's food please start with organic non-GMO seeds and keep it organic (With organic fertilizers, etc.) through the whole cycle.

As Christians we should be the ones paving the way for other folks to do this as well. But sadly it seems that most Christians seem to not even know about the problem or they are in a deep denial of it.

The FDA officially says, "*The health consequences of eating genetically modified organisms are largely unknown*" Well, I guess that means that ingesting a little Roundup with your food MIGHT just be ok as well? (Please understand I am kidding – This would kill you 2 or 3 times over!) However, in fact, if you are eating any GMO food you ARE eating small amounts of roundup not only in residual elements of GMO food but even in it's DNA structure. Just a reminder; most all corn and corn products are now GMO unless labeled USDA ORGANIC.

The facts are; genetically engineered foods have never been shown to be safe to eat in anyway shape or form and will soon have unpredictable consequences to say the least.

Many scientists are worried that the genetically altered foods, once consumed, will pass on their mutant genes to the natural bacterium in the digestive system. This would get real interesting! This could be the beginning of GMO humans. But I guess nothing surprises me anymore.

Once the mutant genes are out of the bag, there is no going back. Genetically modified organisms contaminate existing seeds with their altered material, passing on modified traits to non-target species. This creates a new strain of plant that was never intended even in the laboratory. In North Dakota, recent studies show that 80% of wild canola plants tested contained at least one trans-gene! It is spreading fast! You can't even find organic canola oil; there are not even any safe seeds left! I guess congratulations to Monsanto Company are in order? Help us Lord!

In Japan, a modified bacteria created a new amino acid not found in nature; it was used in protein drinks and before it was recalled it cause severe mental and metabolic damage to hundreds as well as several deaths. Japan banned GMOs after this horrific experience. I can't help but wonder, what will it take for us? What will it take for the country that is leading the way to pushing this stuff on the rest of the world?

In experiments, the organs of rats that ate genetically modified potatoes showed signs of chronic wasting, and female rats fed a diet of herbicide-resistant soybeans gave birth to stunted and sterile pups.

GMOs require massive amounts of pesticides, herbicides and fungicides. These things are poisons, and should not be eaten or allowed to run off into our water supply. But they are, every day, by companies who care far more about the bottom line than they do about your health, or your children's future.

The bottom line is that genetically modified organisms have not been proven in any way to be safe, which is why most of the world's countries have banned these items whose DNA has been genetically engineered.

In America, they aren't even labeled, much less banned, so the majority of the populace has no idea that they are eating lab-created DNA on a daily basis. WELL NOW YOU DO! Just remember, your best defense is to purchase certified organic food, which cannot contain any GMOs, and to tell your friends and loved ones to do the same.

So who is responsible for all this GMO stuff?

The Monsanto Company in conjunction with your wonderful government's FDA is trying hard to push this stuff down our throats. (And they are trying hard to sell it to the rest of the world, even though the rest of the world doesn't want it) And it is not just the FDA. An amazing list of Monsanto employees is found throughout our government. For example, Supreme Court Judge Clarence Thomas was Monsanto's lawyer! (A guy I used to like) The list goes on and on and is too big to list here. Just put in a search for "Monsanto employees in the halls of government" and you will see just what we are up against.

Also, possibly the largest single supporter of Monsanto's evil is the world famous "Do-gooder" Bill Gates! As of this writing, he's already invested $27 million into the Monsanto Company "trying to save the world" It amazes me how someone so smart could be so stupid to not see the disasters of GMO (Or maybe he DOES know what he is doing? Who knows?)

His efforts have led many countries to reject his "charity" due to the high risks, such as: New disease vectors, Mutated pesticide-resistant insects, Resistant "super-weeds" and worst of all, contamination of surrounding non-GMO crops which could eventually wipe out anything from being organic. God help us!

Most people do not realize that genetically engineered foods were only approved in the U.S. because **THE FDA HID 40,000 DOCUMENTS INDICATING THEIR EXTREME TOXICITY!**

Countries around the globe are making it increasingly clear that they're not going to continue to let Monsanto abuse the health of their people and crops without putting up a fight. However, our good ol' USA with the combined forces of Monsanto and the FDA keeps pushing this stuff!

The heart and soul of America are NOT the bad guys of the world but it sure looks like it to the rest of the world thanks to Monsanto! You and I and all citizens of this great country are caught in the middle because of this partnership with evil in our government.

I am reminded of Sodom and Gomorra, but this time the good guys DO outweigh the bad guys. All that is needed is some good old fashioned prayer for forgiveness. And here is the really stupid part: Hardly anyone (ESPECIALLY CHRISTIANS) even knows this evil exists. This is one of the reasons I was compelled to write this book. I know that if Christians became truly aware of this evil within our government they would, at least pray a prayer for forgiveness for this nation and to remove the evil.

So my prayer is, "Lord, please have mercy on us and do not cause us to perish for our ignorance. Please look at the many souls that have been so cleverly deceived by this enemy and have pity on them. We stand on Your word that says:

"If my people, which are called by my name, shall humble themselves, and pray, and seek my face, and turn from their wicked ways; then will I hear from heaven, and will forgive their sin, and will heal their land" - 2 Chronicles 7:14

A close look at the Monsanto Company:

A man with a very dark history named John Francis Queeny (1859-1933) was the founder of The Monsanto Company. He was a Knight of Malta Irish-American ROMAN Catholic serving the Black Pope's University in St Lewis directly. (The "Black Pope" is The Superior General of the Society of Jesus or Jesuits) Queeny founded The Monsanto Company in 1901.

Monsanto is now a US based agricultural and pharmaceutical monopoly; Monsanto Company is a producer of herbicides, prescription pharmaceutical drugs and genetically engineered GMO seeds.

The global Monsanto Corporation has operated sales offices, manufacturing plants, and research facilities in more than 100 countries. They have the largest share of the global GMO crops market. In 2001 its crops accounted for 91% of the total area of GMO crops planted worldwide. Based on 2001 figures

Monsanto was the second biggest seed company in the world, and the third biggest agrochemical company.

Historically Monsanto has been involved with the production of PCBs, DDT, dioxins and the defoliant / chemical weapon 'Agent Orange' (sprayed on American troops and Vietnamese civilians during the Vietnam War). Originally a chemical company, Until the late 1990s Monsanto was a much larger 'life-sciences' company whose business covered chemicals, polymers, food additives and pharmaceuticals, as well as agricultural products.

All of these other chemical business areas have now been de-merged or sold off. Monsanto sold its chemical business in 1997 to build a presence in biotechnology, developing NON-ORGANIC GMO soybeans and corn (classified as a pesticide and banned in the EU) to resist the poisonous effects of its own Roundup herbicide.

Monsanto's key business areas are now agrochemicals, seeds and GMO crops. Monsanto also produced NutraSweet, a GMO sugar substitute. Monsanto recently sold it's GMO bovine growth hormones monopoly to Eli Lilly, and sold it's aspartame (NutraSweet) business to Pfizer.

Monsanto's business is currently run in two parts: Agricultural Productivity, and Seeds and Genomics. The Agricultural Productivity segment includes Roundup herbicide and other agrochemicals, and the Animal Agriculture business. The Seeds and Genomics segment consists of seed companies and related biotechnology traits, and a technology platform based on plant genomics. In reality of course these two segments are inseparable, since the agro-chemicals are becoming increasingly dependent on the seeds segment for sales.

An entire book could be written on the evil history of Monsanto **and I don't want to be the one to write it**! However if you put in a search on your computer with the words: "Monsanto's Dark History" or something like that, you will see stuff that will curl your hair round and round!

Obama has now signed the "Monsanto Protection Act"

From Natural News:

President Barack Obama campaigned on promises to end secret prisons, decriminalize marijuana, balance the budget, honor the Second Amendment and make health care affordable. But what really unfolded was an explosion in the national debt (now $16 trillion and climbing), the signing of the NDAA, a claimed new power to kill any American at any time even on U.S. soil, the use of military drones to murder American children overseas, a full-on assault against the Bill of Rights, a doubling of health insurance rates and the destruction of the U.S. economy.

But that's not all.

Now Obama has signed the "Monsanto Protection Act" into law, stabbing America in the heart yet again and proving that no matter how convincing politicians appear on the campaign trail, they are still sociopathic liars in the end.

The Monsanto Protection Act, part of the HR 933 continuing resolution allows Monsanto to override U.S. federal courts on the issue of planting experimental genetically engineered crops all across the country. Even if those experimental crops are found to be extremely dangerous or to cause a runaway crop plague, the U.S. government now has no judicial power to stop them from being planted and harvested.

As ibtimes.com reports, the bill "effectively bars federal courts from being able to halt the sale or planting of GMO or GE crops and seeds, no matter what health consequences from the consumption of these products may come to light in the future."

GMOs now evade all regulations: America has become a grand Monsanto experiment

A Food Democracy Now petition now states:

With the Senate passage of the Monsanto Protection Act, biotech lobbyists are one step closer to making sure that their new GMO crops can evade any serious scientific or regulatory review.

This dangerous provision, the Monsanto Protection Act, strips judges of their constitutional mandate to protect consumer and farmer rights and the environment, while opening up the floodgates for the planting of new untested genetically engineered crops, endangering farmers, citizens and the environment.

Corporate-government conspiracy is fascism

This new law forces the USDA to automatically approve all GMO planting permits sought by Monsanto and other biotech firms, effectively granting Monsanto dominion over the U.S. government. This is the very definition of fascism, a form of tyrannical government where corporations conspire with the government to destroy or confiscate all rights, powers and assets, leaving the people impoverished and powerless.

51

CHAPTER 2: THE SATANIC ATTACK ON OUR FOOD SUPPLY

What's interesting about this development is that now **even democrats are starting to wake up and see how evil Obama really is.** As ibtimes reports:

"In this hidden backroom deal, Sen. Mikulski turned her back on consumer, environmental and farmer protection in favor of corporate welfare for biotech companies such as Monsanto," Andrew Kimbrell, executive director of the Center for Food Safety, said in a statement. "This abuse of power is not the kind of leadership the public has come to expect from Sen. Mikulski or the Democrat Majority in the Senate."

Of course, for those of us who have been paying attention and warning everyone else about the dangerous power grab taking place under the Obama regime, this is exactly the kind of behavior we expected to see. The Senate has abandoned law. It has abandoned the Constitution, the rights of the People and even due process. We are now living under a corporate fascist tyranny where companies like Monsanto, General Electric and GlaxoSmithKline control the government and dictate policy. They literally write the laws.

This Monsanto Protect Act, says the Center for Food Safety, is "an unprecedented attack on U.S. judicial review of agency actions" and "a major violation of the separation of powers."

But that's what Obama has always been about. He's the president who seized control of all farms, food and livestock across America. He's the guy who claims the power the decide who to assassinate anywhere in America. His administration has routinely conspired with Monsanto to endanger the American people and turn America's croplands into a grand, dangerous genetics experiment.

"Pandora's Box is unlocked, Obama just propped open the lid, and there's no way to cram the evil back in," wrote The Daily Sheeple. "I'm personally pledging at least one article per week about Monsanto, their incestuous relationship with the government, and their toxic grip on agriculture. I urge everyone to raise a deafening public outcry -- every voice adds to the noise that we can create."

So just who is to blame for this bill? It is Senators Barbara Mikulski and Roy Blunt, among others:

The chair of the committee that secretly slipped this provision into the bill was Sen. Barbara Mikulski, an **absolute traitor to America** for allowing the Monsanto Protection Act to become law. She could have stopped it, yet she did nothing to oppose it. She actually helped sneak it into law.

Like nearly all U.S. senators, Mikulski is now operating as an outright **enemy of the People** while selling out to corporate interests who are peddling poison and death.

There is hardly a U.S. senator remaining who respects his or her oath of office. While Senators Rand Paul and Ted Cruz are showing real courage in the face of federal tyranny and oppression -- and Sen. Ron Wyden honestly tries to protect the people of Oregon from outrageous federal aggression -- most senators are now little more than **corporate puppets** who obey the bidding of their masters.

Sickeningly, Sen. Mikulski recently praised the creation of a Harriet Tubman memorial honoring the courage of a woman who stood against tyranny and defended the people by creating the Underground Railroad. Yet Mikulski herself does the exact opposite, selling out to Monsanto and betraying people of all races by overseeing the passage of what is essentially a "judicial nullification power" now granted to a dangerous and truly evil corporation. Her actions in this matter were anti-trade, anti-America, anti-human and anti-justice.

Harriet Tubman, a true American hero, would absolutely shudder at the thought that a U.S. Senator honoring her memory was simultaneously betraying the people of America by handing over extra-judicial powers to a corporation engaged in widespread genetic pollution and agricultural malfeasance.

Harriet Tubman was born a slave and risked her life to lead others to freedom. Sen. Mikulski was born a privileged woman who risked nothing to lead her constituents to corporate slavery. For Mikulski to honor Tubman is an insult to the memory of Tubman and the freedom she stood for.

Missouri Sen. Roy Blunt actively conspired with Monsanto to write the provision!

Mikulski wasn't the only Monsanto sellout in the U.S. Senate, of course: Missouri senator Roy Blunt was also part of the conspiracy to stab America in the heart and poison our food. According to another article on ibtimes.com:

The provision's language was apparently written in collusion with Monsanto. Lawmakers and companies working together to craft legislation is by no means a rare occurrence in this day and age. But the fact that Sen. Roy Blunt, Republican of Missouri, actually worked with Monsanto on a provision that in effect allows them to keep selling seeds, which can then go on to be planted, even if it is found to be harmful to consumers, is stunning.

Who opposed the Monsanto Protection Act? Democratic Senator John Tester. As the NY Daily News reports:

Opposing the inclusion of the rider was Sen. John Tester (D-Mont.), who told Politico that the deal worked out with Monsanto was simply bad policy.

"These provisions are giveaways, pure and simple, and will be a boon worth millions of dollars to a handful of the biggest corporations in this country," Tester said.

Tester, of course, has been the voice of reason on several fronts in recent years, including the so-called Food Safety and Modernization Act of 2010 which granted the FDA vast new powers to terrorize gardeners and farmers across America. Sen. Tester proposed amendments that attempted to protect the freedoms of American farmers, but his efforts were of course thwarted by the evil corporate conspirators who now fill the U.S. Senate chambers.

America is lost...what now?

Voted into office by people whose hearts were filled with hope for real change, Obama now reveals himself to be a sinister serpent of deception who betrays the American people at every opportunity. The Obama Deception is the title of the film released by Alex Jones in 2009. At the time, Jones was ridiculed by Obama supporters who said Obama was their savior and anyone who criticized Obama was a racist.

*Now, four years later, it's obvious that once again **Alex Jones was right** about Obama. Even democrats are increasingly realizing this shocking truth as they watch Obama betray the people of America on issues like GMOs, secret prisons, banker bailouts, due process and marijuana.*

*With deceivers like Obama at the helm, America has been turned over to corporate interests, and the rights and liberties of the People have been eviscerated. The U.S. federal government **no longer represents the interests of the people**. It has become a dominant, dangerous and arrogant machine of oppression and tyranny. It has abandoned law, the*

Constitution and the Bill of Rights. It has violated the very principles upon which this nation was founded and now plays God with our seeds, our food and our future.

These are times of such treachery and betrayal that we cannot even imagine the web of deception being weaved to entrap and destroy truth in America. We the People are being deceived by false media propaganda and told everything is fine while Senators and bureaucrats march us into pits of death while corporate bulldozers stand by to quickly cover up the mass graves.

***The United States government is at WAR with the American people**, and that war is being waged with every poison imaginable: genetic pollution, disinfo propaganda, chemical fluoride poisoning, vaccine lobotomies, chemtrails, psychiatric drugs and twisted mental health initiatives. The battleground for this war is your dinner plate, your tap water, your medicine and your core beliefs. The goal of the war is the complete decimation of all cognitive awareness and the abolition of freedom of thought. Give this a few more years, and the mere utterance of any idea critical of the government will be considered an "act of terrorism" punishable by death.*

End Natural News

OK! So once again maybe we should look to the Traditional American Cowboy and see what he thinks of all this!

I personally think he might say something like this: *"Cowboy up you bunch of wimps! Should we just resign ourselves to the fact that Monsanto, the Biotech Bully of St. Louis, controls the dynamics of the marketplace and public policy?*

Should we seek some kind of practical compromise or "coexistence" between organics and Genetically Modified Organisms (GMOs) like some kind of sissy city dudes?

Should we focus our efforts on crop pollution compensation and "controlled deregulation" of genetically engineered (GMO) crops, rather than demanding an outright ban of GMO's?

*The U.S .has 23 million acres of alfalfa, it is the nation's fourth largest crop. 93% of that alfalfa is still currently **NOT** sprayed with toxic herbicides. This is a good thing and it makes me proud. However, among these, even our organic alfalfa is being polluted from pollinating insects carrying Monsanto's mutant genes. Do you think I want my horses and cows eating that crap?*

*Are we going to sit back and let this happen or are we going to cowboy up and ride into Washington for a **big Pow Wow?***

All this author can really say is, "Whew! I'm glad we are done with this chapter on Monsanto! That was some scary stuff! I feel like washing my hands just after writing about it!"

However, If you want to give these "great folks" at The Monsanto Company a call and let 'em know just how much you appreciate them, here are the contacts and a few facts; *(Oh, and by the way I would appreciate if you do not let them know where you got their security number, I think Monsanto hates me enough already, Thanks for understanding)*

Monsanto Chemical Co. World Headquarters
 800 North Lindbergh Boulevard
St. Louis, Missouri 63167 U.S.A.
Telephone: (314) 694-1000

Fax: (314) 694-6572

http://www.monsanto.com/

Statistics: Public Company

Incorporated: 1933 as Monsanto Chemical Company

Employees: 21,900

Sales: $8.64 billion (1998)

Stock Exchanges: New York, Amsterdam, Brussels, Chicago

Ticker Symbol: MTC

NAIC: 325412 Pharmaceutical Preparations; 325311 Medicinal & Botanical

Manufacturing

Principal Subsidiaries: Calgene Inc. (leader in plant biotech); Asgrow Seed Co.; DEKALB Genetics Corp. (second-largest seed/corn company in the United States); DEKALB Swine Breeders Inc.;Nutrasweet Co. (aspartame) ;Monsanto Agricultural Co.;

G. D. Searle & Co.

CHAPTER 3:
GOD'S HEALTHCARE PLAN

People often ask me, "Do you take any isolated health supplements or vitamins?" Well my answer is simply "No, only whole food and whole herbs"

The facts are most isolated supplements these days are fast becoming nothing more then isolated FDA approved pharma-garbage! I don't like anything isolated. Isolation takes centrifuges and agitators and all kinds of gizmos to separate molecules. Now don't get me wrong, I am not Amish! I know cars and planes aren't in the Bible either but they aren't food and medicine! God was very specific about our food and medicine. It has to be in its whole form the way God made it. Man can't make that! I only trust God's idea for my health. The natural system of whole plants in the form of Tonic Herbs or medicine is so much more effective for specific problems and for pure radiant health that I just can't believe many people don't just get it! I am glad you and I do!

So here is my personal daily practice: (This is not necessarily my advice to you but it works well for me)

First thing every day when I wake up I drink Tulsi Tea and am feeling so great after a cup in the morning! It kind of "clears the cobwebs" out of my brain and within about 15 minutes I can concentrate better and am somehow in a better mood. I have never seen such great results from a simple and good tasting tea before in my life! Tulsi is actually just a type of Basil that grows wild in the foothills of the Himalayas (And conveniently now in our backyard here in Cochise County Arizona) I just started some seeds and they really took off. Strangely the smell and taste of dried Tulsi "tea" reminds me a lot of the taste of a not so healthy drink called "Coca Cola". I have always wondered if it might be one of the original ingredients of Coca Cola that are such a closely guarded secret.

As far as taking any other herbs daily, (Not as medicine but as a daily tonic) my wife takes two herbs and I take three herbs on a regular basis. We both take He Shou Wu (Polygonum muiltiflorum) and Jiao Gu Lan (Gynastemma pentaphyllum) We take a heaping teaspoon of He Shou Wu powder once a day and four droppers twice daily of Jiao Gu Lan Extract.

I also recently started taking Schizandrae (Wu Wei Zi) tincture once a day. I am noticing much better lung energy, more alertness and focus, I don't tend to fall asleep in the chair after work now and I sleep like a rock at night. Considering that this herb has been associated with longevity and is great for the immune system, I will keep taking it!

Also about twice a year we take Ojibwa Tea for two weeks to help clean out any heavy metals we may have accumulated. Oh, and I eat a small handful of Sun Dried Wolfberries almost every day, that's about it!

Now of course on those special days when a very big task is at hand such as having to work all day cutting lots of wood for the winter, I will take Siberian Ginseng tincture for energy.

Also If there is a bit of a flu epidemic around or something, I will be taking Strong Defense capsules (Made from Reshi Mushroom and Astragalus Root Extract) We just don't get sick when we are taking this. I take it when ever I visit someone with the flu and never worry.

And if I ever do feel something like a flu coming on I will take a big "Swig" of Viral Defense twice daily for one or two days. It has never failed me. I have not been sick in over 30 years because of it. At my business (Plant Cures Inc) Viral Defense has quickly become the best seller for return orders as many people know it will stop flu or other infection almost immediately and always like to keep it around. It tastes a little rough so be sure to have a "chaser" handy. Lemonade (The real stuff) works good for this. By the way, Viral Defense can be obtained at PLANTCURES.COM.

I am often asked if I am a strict vegetarian or "vegan". The answer is (Give me a break) NO! We raise cattle, you dummies!" (Not you) We also have chickens and I eat their eggs every other day or so for breakfast. When I don't eat eggs I have a little organic "Seeds N' Nuts" whole grain toast with real whole organic peanut butter and I also cover it with raw honey or this great organic apricot jam my wife makes from our tree. Mmmmm!

Also as a mater of fact (Confession time!) we have a bit of a "Cowboy Diet" going on. We both eat a little too much red meat! (This is one reason I take Jaio Gu Lan and He Shou Wu every day – keeps the cholesterol and HDL/LDL protein binders healthy and has some preventative anti-cancer action)

However, we DO try to make up for it. About twice a week we have meals (Actually, whole days) that are all vegetarian from our own organic garden. The steaks and meat we eat are mostly from animals we know were raised as organically as possible. In the summer, their meat is usually cooked outside on mesquite wood and eaten outdoors as well. I think it is very important to spend as much time living and eating outdoors as possible

Everything is always accompanied with a fresh organic mixed green salad smothered with my wife's home made dressing of Extra Virgin Olive Oil, Balsamic Vinegar and lots of Fresh Crushed Garlic. (There are always lots of onions and tomatoes from our garden in the salad as well)

Another reason I think we are blessed with good health is our habit of eating live cultured yogurt smothered with a variety of organic berries every night. We are addicted!

So what do we do for exercise? I guess a lot when I think about it. First of all we ride our horses almost every day. And in spite of the fact that we live on a small ranch and have many chores with all the animals and weeding and upkeep (While running a large herbal business all day) my wife and I still find time to run a full mile every other day or so.

I am sometimes up at 5:00 AM preparing herbal formulas and answering emails or checking the ranch fence (My wife is often taking care of the garden at this time) and at 5:00 PM I get away from that darn computer and all the packaging then go into "Ranch Mode" and try to maintain this place we call home.

About half the year we also take time to swim everyday in the afternoon (with our dogs) I am only sorry there is not more time in the day! And did I say something about sleep? Wow! Like a rock! However if our dogs bark at something or someone in the night we are up like a private in boot camp running out with flashlights, bibles and guns.

Our life is a hoot! I dearly thank God for it. Every day is a super blessing and I want to reach up and face the sky and just say, THANKS GOD!

But sometimes, just when I look up, the sky looks like a total mess! It just ruins the whole day when all you want to do is praise God as you look up to his wonderful creation.

You have all seen this lately. It is like long trails of white powder start appearing from horizon to horizon They often start in the morning and continue to spread out until the whole sky is a dirty white haze and you begin to feel terrible as your eyes start to burn and you often find yourself coughing and wheezing. The US Weather Service refuses to talk about it and your local TV weather guy really tries hard to keep his job and make excuses for it.

Those ugly white lines in our skies! What is going on?

These "contrails" that turn into "clouds" (Which everybody now calls chemtrails) are a product of the absolute warped brains of those that practice the money grabbing scam of "global warming". Some actually believe in global warming and fear it. They are the pawns, the ones they are counting on to spread the lie as the truth.

These "contrails" are now made up of primarily aluminum nano-particles geared to supposedly reflect the heat back upward. The scientists behind all this take great pride in doing this nonsense and refer to it as aerosol stratospheric geo-engineering. These toxic "clouds" are extremely dangerous to your health and many say this is the greatest crime ever perpetrated on mankind as they have succeeded in ruining the very air we breathe.

What is not clear is what branch of the government is using these planes to do all this and why the government will not admit they are doing it at all. The government has not only been denying this for years but now has the nerve to have developed a sort of "standardized smirk" in their language as an effort to make the public think it is only the "crazies" that would ever DARE to notice this. The only conspiracy surrounding geo-engineering is that government and media refuses to publicly admit what anyone with eyes can see.

The amazingly controlled policy of DENY-DENY-DENY from the government has got the media somehow paralyzed with fear to ever talk about it. Or at least they will not talk about it without passing on that "standardized smirk" to the viewers so their fears (fears of "WHAT?" I am not sure) are pacified.

Our local station in Tucson did just that a few months back. It was so amazingly shameful that comments on the stations "viewers' post" were off the charts with complaints! There was, of course, no comment from Tucson's KGUN channel 9.

However, a month later the aluminum particles got so heavy that the TV station's weather radar would not work. Everyone could see the fake clouds building up so they had to make up an excuse. The TV meteorologist called it "Military Chaff" for purposes of jamming radar as a "training mission"

We know that these persistent contrails contain an amount of aluminum particles that is over 60 times beyond the CDC's legal safe limit and we know they are causing very many new respiratory problems and making many people very sick..

Dr. Russell L Blaylock is a world renowned neurosurgeon, retired from Neurosurgery to devote his full attention to nutritional studies and research. An in-demand guest for radio and TV programs, he lectures extensively to both lay audiences and physicians on nutrition-related subjects. He is the 2004 recipient of the Integrity in Science Award granted by the Weston A Price Foundation and is a member of the editorial board of the Journal of American Physicians and Surgeons, the official publication of the Association of American Physicians and Surgeons. Here is what he has to say about Chemtrails:

"The Internet is littered with stories of "chemtrails" and geoengineering to combat "global warming" and until recently I took these stories with a grain of salt. One of the main reasons for my skepticism was that I rarely saw what they were describing in the skies.

But over the past several years I have noticed a great number of these trails and I have to admit they are not like the contrails I grew up seeing in the skies. They are extensive, quite broad, are laid in a definite pattern and slowly evolve into artificial clouds. Of particular concern is that there are now so many dozens every day littering the skies.

My major concern is that there is evidence that they are spraying tons of nanosized aluminum compounds. It has been demonstrated in the scientific and medical literature that nanosized particles are infinitely more reactive and induce intense inflammation in a number of tissues. Of special concern is the effect of these nanoparticles on the brain and spinal cord, as a growing list of neurodegenerative diseases, including Alzheimer's dementia, Parkinson's disease and Lou Gehrig's disease (ALS) are strongly related to exposure to environmental aluminum.

Nanoparticles of aluminum are not only infinitely more inflammatory, they also easily penetrate the brain by a number of routes, including the blood and olfactory nerves (the smell nerves in the nose). Studies have shown that these particles pass along the olfactory neural tracts, which connect directly to the area of the brain that is not only most effected by Alzheimer's disease, but also the earliest affected in the course of the disease. It also has the highest level of brain aluminum in Alzheimer's cases.

The intranasal route of exposure makes spraying of massive amounts of nanoaluminum into the skies especially hazardous, as it will be inhaled by people of all ages, including babies and small children for many hours. We know that older people have the greatest reaction to this airborne aluminum.

Because of the nanosizing of the aluminum particles being used, home filtering system will not remove the aluminum, thus prolonging exposure, even indoors.In addition to inhaling nanoaluminum, such spraying will saturate the ground, water and vegetation with high levels of aluminum. Normally, aluminum is poorly absorbed from the GI tract, but nanoaluminum is absorbed in much higher amounts. This absorbed aluminum has been shown to be distributed to a number of organs and tissues including the brain and spinal cord. Inhaling this environmentally suspended nanoaluminum will also produce tremendous inflammatory reaction within the lungs, which will pose a significant hazard to children and adults with asthma and pulmonary diseases.

I pray that the pilots who are spraying this dangerous substance fully understand that they are destroying the life and health of their families as well. This is also true of our political officials. Once the soil, plants and water sources are heavily contaminated there will be no way to reverse the damage that has been done.

Steps need to be taken now to prevent an impending health disaster of enormous proportions if this project is not stopped immediately. Otherwise we will see an explosive increase in neurodegenerative diseases occurring in adults and the elderly in unprecedented rates as well as neurodevelopmental disorders in our children. We are already seeing a dramatic increase in these neurological disorders and it is occurring in younger people than ever before".

Russell L. Blaylock, M.D.

Visiting Professor Biology

Belhaven University

Theoretical Neurosciences Research, LLC

But here comes the fun part! What would the Traditional American Cowboy say about "chemtrails"? Well, after riding with a few of you, I was not surprised to hear the words, *"My, don't them things make a pretty sunset!"* However this wonderful innocence of having no clue there could be such evil in the world may be the way God wants it for many of us. And if that is the case I apologize for even bringing this up in this book but I must tell you the truth. I felt this really needs to be exposed. I know these artificial clouds with their aluminum particle base are a huge factor in harming our health. I pray daily that God will soon send someone who will be able to break through this fog of denial to where this evil practice is exposed to the public and banned forever.

What does the Bible say about using drugs as medicine?

The very first place the word "medicine" is used in the Bible is in Proverbs 17:22 and it says, "A merry heart doeth good, like a medicine. The very next text listed in the concordance under medicine is found in EZ. 47:12, "The fruit thereof shall be for meat and the leaf thereof for medicine.

In the New Testament, it really gets down to the nitty-gritty!

Strong's exhaustive concordance of the Bible, which lists every word in the Bible, lists the word "sorcery" as word #5332 and tells us that it is translated from the original Greek word "Pharmacia" It gives the definition as: a drug i.e. a spell-giving potion, A druggist or pharmacist, is called a prmakon meaning a poisoner.

The Bible says that "sorcery" (the use of poisonous drugs) has deceived all nations. "For by thy sorceries (Pharmacia) were all nations deceived. And in her was found the blood of prophets, and of saints, and of all that were slain upon the earth". (Rev. 18:23,24)

You can also look in Webster's 2nd Collegiate Dictionary published in 1980 under the word "pharmaceutical." The definition reads: "pharmaceutical" the practice of witchcraft or the use of poison.

In a response to my posting of this on the internet, a "Christian pharmacist" emailed me trying to defend the pharmaceutical industry and proclaimed: *"There's a reason that the word "Pharmacea" is often translated "sorcery". He went on to say, "Here is a quote from Vine's Expository Dictionary of New Testament Words, regarding this word: "In sorcery, the use of drugs, whether simple or potent, was generally accompanied by incantations and appeals to occult powers, with the provision of various charms, amulets, etc., professedly designed to keep the applicant or patient from the attention and power of demons, but actually to impress the applicant with the mysterious resources and powers of the sorcerer." This is from Thayer's Greek Lexicon, defining the word "Pharmacea" as: "One who prepares or uses magical remedies".*

I wrote him back with the following reply:

"You are absolutely right! And the evil spells, incantations, misdirection, etc, you are talking about is, in fact, exactly how the drug industry of today works.

Think about it; just what do you think all those drug pushing commercials really are? Are they not modern-day incantations to hypnotically make you take drugs? This is in fact, witchcraft and sorcery at its most refined moment in history! It is finely tuned, beautifully orchestrated, and masterfully executed.

The "Master of Evil" is also a master of disguise and deception and he is not going to make it look like a "Harry Potter episode" when evil spells are worked and put into action in the first century. We are not limited to our imagination's concepts of "fairyland witches and sorcerers" Wake up! This is genuinely real modern day evil. Thanks for the letter though.

Almost prophetically Thomas Jefferson gave us this warning: "If people let government decide what foods they eat and what medicines they take, their bodies will soon be in as sorry a state as are the souls of those who live under tyranny." Remember, this statement was made about 100 years before there ever even was an FDA!

What really gets me is just how "smart" these "pharma-geek scientists" are! It is EXACTLY like a bratty little child talking back to God The Father saying, *"We don't like what you gave us for medicine. It is dumb. We are smart. We are going to make our own medicine. We will separate one of your molecules at a time. You have to let us borrow some coal-tar you made to get the molecules from though IT'S NOT FAIR IF YOU DON'T! We will also make laws to make sure no one gets your stupid herbs for medicine"* - This sounds very much like The Tower of Babel to me. Most of you know how that story ended.

A quick reality check: Now please don't panic and think this book is saying the equivalent of, *"You are all going to hell because you have taken an aspirin now and then or give one to your child!"* **Nor is this book saying that if you are old and have been taking a lot of Pharma-drugs for a long time that you should just suddenly stop taking them! (This could be very dangerous)**

Just remember, If you want to get off all your drugs please first PRAY. Then go slowly and get advice form a natural healthcare practitioner first. Though rare, drug withdrawals could kill you if not done slowly! Does that make you wonder why you ever started taking them? Well we know it was the way you were brought up; believing that we should always take the "Good Doctor's advice" It was really not your fault and God understands all of this. However you will always live a longer healthier life taking only natural food and medicine because this was God's plan for us in our very creation.

So should we ever see an MD? Well of course! If you have a traumatic injury from a car accident, gunshot wounds, broken bones, have arrows sticking through your head or you need a cleft palate fixed, (Come on, use a little common sense) by all means see an MD (The key word is "traumatic injury")

However, and this is a big however, (It is also just my opinion) If you have a health related problem such as high blood pressure, cholesterol, heart arrhythmias, flu, viral infection or anything that is not an injury, then going to an MD will most likely wind up with a doctor causing you to take very dangerous drugs. You also just gave up all your other choices and freedoms the moment you walked into his office.

This is exactly what it has come down to now. Nothing whole and natural is ever even considered any more as a means of treatment. It has to be synthetic and therefore always poisonous FDA approved drugs. Do you actually believe the FDA is looking out for our health? (A whole other book could be written on this)

These drugs go against every natural law in our God-created body as far as how our liver, kidneys, heart and other organs will respond. Also our bodies become quickly enslaved to it.

Sure drugs may do the trick of lowering blood pressure or reducing cholesterol or keeping you from getting pregnant or God only knows what else but does that mean they are ultimately good for your health? Definitely not! Your body will began trying to reject any synthetic food or drug immediately and at some point if your body can not reject them, your organs will weaken or fail from trying so hard to reject the drug.

Just because the symptom (high blood pressure, high cholesterol, or whatever) is adjusted, it does not have a thing to do at all with our actual health! Why can't the general public see this? It only proves that a poison has succeeded in temporarily altering a symptom by a force. A deadly toxic force none the less. They never did one thing to try to help the actual balance of health in the body to have a part in correcting the problem.

Oh, and those "chemtrails"? Well all I can say is start asking questions and take pictures. Call your local TV stations and let them see your videos. Something is really going on that is somehow hidden by the media from the public's very eyes even though we can all see it! It does not make sense how they can keep denying it and the media keeps giving them a free pass to deny it. I personally think this is just another classic satanically controlled thing.

The reason I say this is due to all the un-explained facts of why and how this can be kept so hidden while it is right in front of our eyes. They certainly are not common jet-contrails. That much is for sure. I wish I had more answers. God I pray you give us clarity on this and expose it once and for all that it be banned forever!

What about all those "cancer screenings" they always want us to have?

First let's take a look at these five basic facts:

1: The cancer business is absolutely huge being funded by "research drives" with "pink ribbon walks" and all sorts of boloney always claiming that a cure is "just around the corner" This is one of the most successful scams in history! Don't buy it!

2: In reality, the last thing any of these chemo companies like Monsanto, GlaxoSmithKline, DuPont and others want is a "cure". A real cure, of which I am sure there are many, (natural cures) would destroy all of this wonderful income and they would be flat out of business. This is the reason that when someone is cured of cancer by herbs the cure is not allowed to be published anywhere. They can actually arrest you if you even publish it on the internet. What happened to freedom of speech? They say by publishing (especially on a website) that you are claiming in an "advertisement" that you have a "new drug" and thereby must pay the FDA millions of dollars to even consider this new drug. Of course they would never consider it unless they could be in on the profit. And no profit could be made because herbs can not be patented. However I guess Monsanto COULD claim a patent on a genetically modified herb (Now that is really scary)

3: The media is powerful and has already convinced the average person that *What ever is discussed on TV with professional doctors must be good advice*" How dare we even try to argue?

4: The Chemo drugs made by Monsanto and others have an expensive price tag and these companies MUST find a way to get business. It is a known fact they will stop at nothing until the public is convinced.

5: Most doctors are easily trained in medical schools (mostly built and sponsored by drug companies) to believe that the drug protocol is the "word of god" in medical practice. So when people are told to "Ask their doctors" from TV commercials the drug companies (drug pushers in reality) get 100% assurance that their drugs will be bought and administered. It is quite a well thought out scam when you think about it!

Space does not permit me to comment on all the scams associated with the cancer industry as this is not at all a book on cancer. However, the "breast cancer scam" is worth mentioning here. Most other countries other than the US have done studies on the dangers of breast mammography.

I have said this before and will say it again, I am a patriot, I love this country, but it seems our government is either the cruelest, non-caring, death dealing, genocidal of any in the world when it comes to drugs, medical procedures, the corruption of our food supply, and our general health. I personally do not know if it is stupidity or diabolical. Take your pick! Either one is dangerous.

As an example, The Nordic Cochrane Center points out that screening actually creates breast cancer patients out of healthy women who would never have developed symptoms. Treatment of these healthy women increases their risk of dying from heart disease and, yes, cancer itself.

According to the Nordic Cochrane Center; *"It therefore no longer seems reasonable to attend for breast cancer screening. In fact, by avoiding going to screening, a woman will lower her risk of getting a breast cancer diagnosis."*

Radiation risks are some four-fold greater for the 1 to 2 percent of women who are silent carriers of the A-T (ataxia-telangiectasia) gene; by some estimates this accounts for up to 20 percent of all breast cancers diagnosed annually.

You really don't have to be a nuclear physicist and physician to understand that mammograms (x-rays) cause cancers, BUT IT HELPS! Dr. Gofman is a nuclear physicist and a medical doctor and this is his conclusion. *"Mammography is a perfect example of modern medicine "putting the cart before the horse." Although there is no evidence that it saves lives, that is exactly what everyone is led to believe"*

He went on to say, *"Breast cancer is a largely PREVENTABLE disease, and we reach that good news because of our finding that a large share of recent and current breast cancer in the United States is CERTAINLY due to past medical irradiation of the breasts with x-rays - at all ages, including infancy and childhood. Much of today's radiation dosage is preventable, without any interference with necessary diagnostic radiology, and hence many future breast cancers need not occur."*

Professor Samuel Epstein concurs with the risks mammograms and x-rays in general pose for the unknowing patient: *"X-rays are carcinogenic. The more X-rays you submit to and the greater the dose, the greater is your risk of cancer... Whatever you may be told, refuse routine mammograms to detect early breast cancer, especially if you are pre-menopausal. The X-rays may actually increase your chances of getting cancer.... Very few circumstances, if any, should persuade you to have X-rays taken if you are pregnant. The future risks of leukemia to your unborn child, not to mention birth defects, are just not worth it."*

The facts are mammography screening is a profit-driven technology posing risks compounded by total unreliability. Radiation from routine mammography poses high cumulative risks of initiating and promoting breast cancer. How much risk you ask? The routine practice of taking four films of each breast annually results in approximately 1 rad (radiation absorbed dose) exposure which is about 1,000 times greater than that from a chest x-ray. This is compounded by the fact that screening mammography poses much higher significant and cumulative risks of breast cancer for pre-menopausal women.

1,000 times that of a chest x-ray??? Wow! On a personal note, I would never allow even one chest-x-ray on my self. If I suspected pneumonia, tuberculosis, or even lung cancer I would just treat what ever disease I suspected naturally with an appropriate herbal therapy and my chances of a complete recovery would be at least as good as any allopathic profit driven treatment. Plus (And this is a big plus) no harm would be done to my body and even if I died, I would suffer no side effects from anything and be on my way home to Jesus with relatively no pain before death. What would I gain by going the pharma / medical way?

CHAPTER 4:
LIFE WITHOUT PRESCRIPTION DRUGS

The Cholesterol Myth: A lie to get you hooked!

I don't know about you but I am getting awfully tired of seeing people lied to by their doctors as a way to push the deadly drug protocol of statin drugs. If you believe all the hype from Pharmaceutical Reps and TV commercials then you will also believe that the whole reason our livers make cholesterol is simply to give us a heart attack sometime down the road! Well that is certainly not the reason God made MY liver!

As you will see, there is no "good" or "bad" cholesterol. This is a lie made up by the drug companies to push drugs. The truth is CHOLESTEROL IS JUST CHOLESTEROL. (A fatty, waxy chemical substance created in the liver used in the construction of our cells) We all desperately need this wonderful substance called cholesterol to make all our hormones and in fact reproduce any cells in our bodies.

The statin drugs they will try to push at you will cause your liver to shut down its natural process of making this wonderful life giving substance! Think about it. Is this what you really want to do to yourselves?

It is a fact that our brains are largely made up of cholesterol and therefore Alzheimer's and many other disorders are many times a result of people lacking a healthy amount of cholesterol. There is more and more cases of Alzheimer's popping up all the time. And more and more research data shows this is largely due to statin drugs shutting down livers and stopping cholesterol production!

HERE ARE THE FACTS; LDL or so called "bad cholesterol" Is not a type of cholesterol at all! It is in fact just a protein. Low density lipoprotein to be exact. LDL is a binding protein that is necessary to carry cholesterol to the whole body from the liver as needed because the waxy cholesterol is not soluble in our watery blood. Therefore it needed a binder which God provided. This is all LDLs and HDLs are. This not at all a type of cholesterol.

HDL is the other protein binder designed to help carry the used-up cholesterol back to the liver. It is not to "get rid of" cholesterol as the pharma-medical system would have you believe but to recycle it so we can use it again and again. The simple facts are we need all three! Cholesterol, LDL protein and HDL protein are all essential to a normal functioning body.

The only "bad" cholesterol is cholesterol that has become oxidized and the only way to undo this oxidation is by feeding our bodies with anti-oxidant rich foods and herbs.

Good healthy cholesterol is made of large round particles that flow through the blood easily. When a sample test is done there is not as much room (In parts per million) for big healthy particles so the count will often be lower. Sometimes cholesterol particles can be smaller but still healthy and round and flowing easy. This is just our personal body chemistry and does not mean you are about to have a heart attack or stroke. This is why the "Cholesterol numbers game" is really just a scam to sell drugs.

However if you have an unhealthy oxidized form of cholesterol causing the particles to be small and irregularly shaped (And thereby easy to bind up in your arteries) Then you should seek a better diet and an herbal formula to correct this.

Please remember these facts: LDL is a protein blood-binder to mix cholesterol with the blood going to our body cells from the liver. HDL is a protein blood-binder to mix cholesterol with the blood going back to the liver. And **CHOLESTEROL IS JUST CHOLESTEROL!**

Remember, the only "bad" cholesterol is that which has become oxidized and corrupt with plaque and the only way to undo this oxidation and plaque is by feeding our bodies with anti-oxidant rich foods and herbs that help clean-up the blood. It is one of the easiest things for diet and proper herbs to do.

You can have a lot of fun with those drug pushing doctors (If you can stand to be around them) that keep telling you that you have different types of cholesterol. Some may be so brainwashed from the lies of the drug companies they will be willing to bet! Be sure to have some proof (Easy to find) from a medical manual like "Merck" hidden in your pocket. (Please be advised that gambling is probably illegal in your state)

Or better yet, do as I do and just don't even go to doctors at all unless you are in a horrible car wreck or have another one of those pesky arrows sticking through your head. (I hate it when that happens)

Is it safe to even "HAVE" a doctor these days?

Wow, that is quite a question and who would have ever thought it would even have to come up as a question?

Well please forgive me if I sound like I am ranting and raving (I probably am) but I am going to be as bold and honest as I can and answer it very simply.

The answer is: Only if the doctor is used strictly for injuries to the body or only if the doctor does not believe in EVER prescribing any pharmaceutical drugs. I realize the non-use of Pharmadrugs narrows it down to almost zero but this is the only way I can answer this question truthfully.

Would I use a doctor if I had a broken leg? Yes. Would I use a doctor if I was sick? Good Lord, NO! Herbs have stronger antibiotic and antiviral effects than any drugs do and they don't compromise your immune system or cause other problems when you take them.

Would I use a doctor if I had a heart problem? NO! Herbs such as Dan Shen can correct so many heart problems without any danger.

Would I use a doctor if I had high blood pressure? NO! Herbs can help this easily.

Would I use a doctor if I was mangled up in a car wreck? Yes by all means!

Do I believe in check-ups by a doctor? My Lord, No! That is the best way to be lied to. (Usually *un-willingly* lied to out of medical indoctrination similar to catholic "dogma") It is also the best way to be subject to dangerous screening or to be told you have cancer due to the very common occurring *false positive* test results. Upwards of 100,000 false positive diagnoses are caught each year and up to 1,000,000 each year are estimated to have "slipped by" sentencing these poor victims to death by chemotherapy. God forgive us!

By the way I believe everyone goes through some sort of cancer from time to time and their immune system normalizes it on it's own as long as you are getting proper nutrition from non-GMO food. If you are "LUCKY" enough to see a doctor when this is going on you can sure have your life ruined fast from chemo drugs. Cancers can always be helped with health, herbs and nutrition better and faster than with poison anyway. Oh, but that isn't the "NORM" is it?

The "NORM" that we have been forced into has everything to do with the corporate pharmaceutical owned media's push on drugs reminding you to always "Ask your doctor" **We have never been duped so much in all of history!**

Since when do we need to ask a doctor anything other than *"Did you get the bullet out yet, doc?"* Why is it "normal" to have our blood pressure or cholesterol or prostates monitored? Why is it "normal" to get "breast exams" Well that answer is simple: It is normal because drugs became very big business when they gained control over our media and most people bit on this evil lie, hook line and sinker so here we are! OK, thanks for listening; I'm through ranting and raving now!

Now just before we get into the various herbs and whole healing energy of God's plants as medicine, I think we need to first cover a shortcut to healing that makes all else seem insignificant......

How To Freely Heal The Sick Through The Name Of Jesus

I grew up in a Christian family and since early childhood I can still hear the echo of the words, *"Lord, guide the doctor's hands in the healing of "Brother So n' so" that he will make a speedy recovery"* The prayer is ended by saying, "In the name of Jesus, Amen"

Now please don't get me wrong, this is not a bad prayer at all! Most doctors can really use our prayers if we put ourselves into their hands. Also by earnestly and truly praying in the name of Jesus, we know the prayer "got to God" However in praying for God to guide the doctors hands, are we not first putting our faith in the medical system and then secondly into Gods hands?

Well before we get into how to pray specifically for healing of the sick let's take a look at the power of prayer, faith and the power of the very name of Jesus:

First of all, prayer through any other name than Jesus is absolutely powerless (unless you consider the power to really screw yourself up which can happen easily by praying in any other name)

I feel so bad when I see articles by doctors and scientists proclaiming that they have now "proven" that prayer works. They go on to say things like, "Whoever or whatever you perceive god to be, there is a mind-body connection that takes place when one prays" In reality they are making excuses for those that have sincerely prayed in the name of Jesus and have had true miraculous healing. This just wouldn't line up with there "god of medical science".

Many good well meaning pastors will often say that we serve a Supernatural God. Well, I would have to say that statement is both true and yet <u>NOT</u> true. Let me explain: Sure, the power of prayer is super and stands out as no other power on earth does and it is "not of this world" (speaking of a totally secular world) but when I look at the way Jesus himself taught us to pray it becomes as natural as it can be and it is just as much of earth as it is of heaven.: ....*Thy kingdom come, thy will be done on EARTH as it is in heaven....*

So why is prayer in the name of Jesus so powerful?

Well. Let's start at the beginning: This is sometimes a hard concept for some and yet so very simple for others but here it is: God is and was always here! He was not created because he did not need to be created. Also when we speak of God we are speaking of the Holy trinity as well. In the beginning was the Word (Who was Jesus) and the Word was with God and the Word was God. This has been in place forever and no part of it (Including Jesus) was ever created by anyone. He was simply always here. However the angels, including Satan (along with us humans) ARE created beings. Created by God!

(Some religious cults actually want you to believe that Jesus was created. They aren't specific about "who" created Him but they say it happened on another planet! In this way they try to convince you that Jesus and Satan are "spiritual brothers")

Now Jesus, of course, did come to earth as God's final sacrifice to us. And yes, He was born to earth by way of a virgin named Mary.

Remember Jesus was God's only beloved son that had always been with Him in heaven. That is exactly why it was and is the greatest sacrifice that could ever happen: God (In the form of *The Son*) came to earth to become man as well as God for a short time. The reason he had to be born of a human was so He could, indeed, become man!

When we look at the awesome power against all of Satan's forces and realize that all we have to do is pray in His name (Much like a "power of attorney") we began to understand just how powerful it is!

His name is so powerful because the name "Jesus" immediately causes all of Satan's forces to tremble with fear knowing that Jesus himself is the very word of God that created all things. The following verses show this:

John 1:1 In the beginning was the Word, and the Word was with God, and the Word was God. 2. He was in the beginning with God. 3. All things were made through Him, and without Him nothing was made that was made. 9. That was the true Light which gives light to every man who comes into the world. 10. He was in the world, and the world was made through Him, and the world did not know Him. 12. But as many as received Him, to them He gave the right to become children of God, even to those who believe in His name. 14. And the Word became flesh and dwelt among us, and we beheld His glory, the glory as of the only begotten of the Father, full of grace and truth.

Revelation 19:13 He was clothed with a robe dipped in blood, and his name is called the Word of God. 16. And He has on His robe and on His thigh a name written: KING OF KINGS AND LORD OF LORDS.

Healing the sick in the name of Jesus was actually a commandment from Jesus:

Jesus sent out the 12 Apostles telling them to, "Go rather to the lost sheep of Israel, as you go, preach this message: The Kingdom of Heaven is near, heal the sick, raise the dead, cleanse those who have leprosy, drive out demons. Freely you have received, freely give." Matthew 10:6-8. Later Jesus sent out the 72 with the same commission when He instructed them, "Heal the sick who are there tell them the Kingdom of God is near you." Luke 10:9.

So how do we heal the sick in the name of Jesus today?

First of all remember that Jesus is the same yesterday, now and forever. Next remember that all of Satan's forces tremble at the very sound of His name. So boldly with faith, open your mouth and pray with the authority over Satan in the name of Jesus! If you have been truly born again, lay both hands on the sick and let the Holy Spirit that lives in you flow through you!

Jesus has given you the power! In John 14:12 Jesus says, " *Most assuredly, I say to you, he who believes in Me, the works that I do he will do also; and greater works than these he will do, because I go to My Father. 13. And whatever you ask in My name, that I will do, that the Father may be glorified in the Son. 14. If you ask anything in My name, I will do it.* So never think you do not have the power to heal the sick in the name of Jesus!

We must also remember we are praying for the sick, not the doctor or the doctor's work! It is very easy for us to try to sort of "help God" or second guess Him as we put or faith in the medical system first. The reason we don't want to pray for the doctor's work is simply that the Holy Spirit may not even want that doctor involved in the healing.

God knows whose hands to use when He wants to. He may possibly use a doctor's hands but most of us just don't have the faith to see that He may not want a doctor's hands any ware NEAR the one you are praying for! Remember, if it is not a traumatic injury (broken bone, large cut or other injury) and it is a disease, a regular doctor will do what he is trained to do which is push the pharmaceutical system's drugs at the patient. The Pharmaceutical industry (As you will see in the next chapter) is one of the most deadly and satanic forces of this world.

(If you pray sincerely God will let you know) This is why we just pray for the sick and stand back and let God do his wonderful work.

Speak the name of Jesus out loud and boldly as you pray!

Don't be afraid to boldly and loudly use the name of Jesus as you pray. It is good if you often say "In the name of Jesus" out loud while you are praying and not just at the end of your prayer. Satan and all his demons must hear you use the name of Jesus. Let them hear it! (Maybe someone in the next room needs to hear it as well) so don't be afraid to speak it out loud.

Remember you have been given the power to heal in His name. The power is NOT from you, it is from Jesus but it flows through you and this is why we say, "You have been given the power" You are just a vessel for delivering this power but you have the awesome responsibility as a vessel to be filled with it and then "pour it out" on the sick. Remember this as you lay hands on that person. You are praying with the authority over Satan to heal and deliver in the precious name of Jesus.

With this kind of powerful prayer in mind as *the first aid we must always use before ever applying any physical thing to healing,* let's take a look at some genuine God given Herbal Medicine:

What herbs did the cowboys use for general health?

I am sure I don't have to remind you that letting drug pushers get you "hooked" on anything they push on TV is just not the cowboy way! In fact I want us to take a look at the history of the cowboys who were one of the main cultures in this country that proved that God's idea of medicine works best and keeps us healthy at the same time:

The culture of the American Cowboy and the use of herbs have widely crossed paths with the American Indian and also with the Mexican cowboys or "Vaqueros". Much of the knowledge of herb-use was also brought in from the "old country" of each cowboy's own heritage.

There is also some major influence from the Chinese due to the Chinese railroad workers who brought their Chinese Medicine with them. They often crossed paths with the cowboy or rancher that was always looking out for the health of his crew. If you were lucky they shared a bit of their knowledge of herbal medicine with you and maybe even gave you some Chinese herbal pills to try.

This incredible mix of medicinal knowledge that fell upon the American cowboy actually inspired one of the best medical systems this country ever had. They were called "The Eclectic Physicians". In fact, this Eclectic Medical System almost caught on big in this country and would have likely been our safe and wholesome American standard of medicine if not shot down by the newly formed A.M.A. (American Medical Association) out of Boston who's efforts to stop all natural herb remedies prevailed and finally won.

"Regular white man's medicine" at the time made extensive use of purges with calomel and other **mercury-based remedies**, as well as extensive bloodletting. (Both of these kinds of practices proved to be not only disastrous but quite "insane" as they killed many more people than they ever helped) Eclectic medicine was a direct reaction as an alternative to those bizarre practices.

In 1915, there were 12,000 Eclectic physicians and 14,000 Homeopathic physicians in practice in the US. During that time there were 8 accredited Eclectic schools, and 9 Homeopathic schools all producing students that sat for the various state boards and took the same tests as everyone else!

By 1935, there remained only 1 eclectic school, and 2 homeopathic schools. By 1940, ALL private medical schools had vanished and ONLY "standard practice" medicine ("allopaths") survived. This was a sad time for the health of America!

But let's get back to the individual heroic medicinal herbs used by the American cowboys: The different regions of the country offered different herbs that were available and growing near by. However, much of the cowboy's herbal medicine came from the Southwest. This includes a vast amount of cattle country including Texas, New Mexico, Utah, Arizona, California, Nevada, Mexico and even parts of Oklahoma and Colorado.

Chaparral: (Larrea tridentata), "Greasewood" or "creosote bush"

Chaparral is perhaps the "King of the Cowboy Herbs" Many camp cooks carried this in the form of a tincture as an important part of there medical supplies.

A tincture, by the way, is a liquid herb extract made by covering the herb with 40% grain alcohol (Such as 80 proof whiskey, vodka or gin) for two weeks then pouring and straining the liquid into a bottle. These tinctures are powerful and will last for many years.

We have all seen Chaparral growing. In some areas it is all you see growing on the desert floor for miles. It is a bush growing up to 10 ft tall covered with small green leaves and has little yellow flowers sometimes depending on the rain. It has a very strong smell and when it rains in the desert you can smell it for many miles.

Chaparral is very common in all of the Southwest. It is also known as "Greasewood" and "Creosote Bush" This herb was a favorite of the Mexican Vaqueros and was used by all the Indian tribes in the region. The American cowboy quickly adopted the use of this herb after seeing how man and beast were healed internally and externally by this amazing plant.

Its uses are legion and there are countless stories of horses (And cowboys) being gored by bulls and surviving by the use of Chaparral powder dusted into there wounds. There are also countless stories of bullets being removed with nothing but Chaparral tincture used as an antiseptic leaving perfect healing.

It has been successfully used against skin fungus, many bacterial infections, (Including dental and urinary tract infections) stopping putrid infections from forming in wounds, and is helpful in Arthritis due to its anti-inflammatory actions.

Chaparral is clearly shown to have a very high antioxidant content, which can protect one against the cell damage which leads to cancer. Some studies on laboratory rats suggest that chaparral actually does inhibit the growth of tumors, while the treated animals survived significantly longer than the ones in the control group.

One of the reasons for this is the fact that Chaparral contains a natural chemical identified as Nordihydroguaiaretic acid. In the Merck Manual, a highly regarded medical book, this chemical is listed as an anti-oxidant, and its therapeutic category is an "anti-neoplastic". Broadly, an anti-neoplastic is defined as "an agent that prevents the development, growth and proliferation of malignant cells". Yep, cancer!

Though all this "anti-cancer stuff" is interesting, this is not at all what the American Cowboys used Chaparral for. It was mostly used against infection simply because it worked and it worked well! In the 1950's Chaparral became know as the "Penicillin of the desert" or even "Cowboy "Penicillin" Besides, there just wasn't much cancer around back when the camp cook carried only whole natural ingredients.

Back in those days "white sugar" was more of a light brown as was the "white flour" because they did not have the processing and refining methods of today such as running the sugar through bone-black which is a known carcinogenic. Cancer was much harder to find in those days!

However it is very interesting (and very embarrassing to the American Medical establishment) that the BBC has no problem exposing what would never reach the media in our own country. Below is a reprint from an article by the BBC or British Broadcasting Company:

BBC Reports on Beneficial Cancer Treatment Based on Native American Tradition - Ancient remedy 'shrinks cancer'

An ancient Native American treatment for cancer has been shown to have a beneficial effect despite skepticism from the medical establishment.

Chaparral, an evergreen desert shrub, has long been used by native Americans to treat cancer, colds, wounds, bronchitis, warts, and ringworm.

But experts dismissed its worth, and warned it could be dangerous.

Now researchers at the Medical University of South Carolina have shown an extract may shrink some tumors.

Chaparral tea was widely used in the US as an alternative anti-cancer agent from the late 1950s to the 1970s. However, the American

Cancer Society said there was no proof that it was an effective treatment for cancer - or any other disease.

And the US Food and Drug Administration warned against its use after research showed it could damage the liver and the kidneys.

However, initial results from the latest study show that an extract of the shrub appears not only to be safe, but to have a positive effect.

The researchers tested a refined extract taken from chaparral called M4N.

They injected it into the tumors of eight patients with advanced head and neck cancer that had not responded to other forms of treatment. The trial was primarily designed to test whether the extract was safe. The results were encouraging - patients seemed to tolerate it well, and there was no evidence of the serious liver damage previously associated with chaparral use.

However, the study also produced some evidence that the extract had begun to shrink the tumors.

I personally have used Chaparral very successfully for many things. I had let my teeth get very bad as a young man. My teeth were full of mercury from many fillings. (Myself nor my parents did not know how dangerous mercury was at that time in the 1960's)

As I got older, I would just basically let my teeth "rot" until I could easily remove them by myself. However there was an important difference: Though my teeth were rotting away, there was no painful abscessing. This was because I kept squirting Chaparral tincture into the "would be" painful area with an eye dropper which stopped the putrid infection from forming while causing an anti-inflammatory action reliving the pain as well.

The teeth would just fall out painlessly. Soon all the mercury laden teeth had left me. The only ones that survived were the ones that had never been exposed to mercury and these teeth (Though few unfortunately) are all healthy.

As another example we had a dog that was gored deep by the tusk of a Javelina. Even when a dog gets an anti-biotic from a vet for this, the dog often does not make it. We happened to have a jar of dried Chaparral powder so we just packed it into the open wound. (Never took her to a vet or used any standard antibiotics) By the second day she was feeling great and full of energy. The wound completely healed and there was never a problem

I once met an old Indian man (A Mescalero Apache) that was still driving his 1964 Buick Wildcat at the age of 105. (He showed me his driver's license proving his age) We had some great discussions and I could have listened to him for hours but the part I remember best is when he said "I have drunk a cup of Chaparral tea every day of my life since the age of 15".

I could go on and on about Chaparral but will need to make room here for other cowboy herbs.

Yellow Dock or "Curled Dock"

This is a fairly common weed that is found all over the world. Yellow Dock has a long history of use amongst the early cowboys and Indians.

First of all the young leaves are a very good pot herb and it was always looked forward to as a healthy and delicious side-dish to beans and tortillas. The camp cook always kept an eye out for it.

It is very rich in iron and other minerals and the root turned out to be a very useful medicine, especially on the long cattle drives.

The root is best known as a gentle and safe laxative, less "radical" than rhubarb in its action but very effective so it was particularly useful in the treatment of mild constipation. (This occurred a lot out on the trail)

This yellow rooted plant has valuable cleansing properties and is useful for treating a wide range of skin problems. It was also used in piles, bleeding of the lungs, various blood complaints and also chronic skin diseases.

Externally, the root can be mashed and used as a poultice and salve, or dried and used as a dusting powder, on sores, ulcers, wounds and various other skin problems. In fact, yellow dock has proved to be an outstanding medication for skin problems like weeping eczema, psoriasis (a chronic disease of the skin consisting of itchy, dry, red patches, usually affecting the scalp or arms and legs)

Yellow Dock is effective in activating clogged blood and lymph. In addition, Yellow Dock can extract toxins out of tissues and also ensure their removal from the body. In fact, the herb can be used wherever there is blockage, heat and irritation.

Women used Yellow Dock for healing unbalanced menstrual cycles, heavy bleeding during periods, menstrual pain and to dissolve fibroids in the uterus and breasts.

Yellow Dock roots are extremely rich in iron content and are, therefore, an exceptional medication for anemia (low hemoglobin content in blood). In fact when you first pull Yellow Dock out of the ground you can often see yellow-orange iron oxide clinging to the roots. It is this plants ability to attract the iron that is most beneficial in curing anemia. (This ability is transferred to the patient via the liver)

You can also get a good amount of iron from the plant itself but the effect it has on your liver causing you to better absorb iron and other minerals is amazing. When you take Yellow Dock and then feed your body iron rich foods like Black Strap Molasses your blood will be back to normal in a few weeks.

"Yellow Dock Syrup" was a wonderful remedy for both anemia and for alleviating problems of the upper respiratory system like emphysema. Here is how it was made:

Take a pint of distilled water and boil half pound of yellow dock root in it until the liquid is diminished to a meager cupful. Sieve the liquid and throw away the boiled root. Add half a cup dark honey half a cup blackstrap molasses and one teaspoon of pure maple syrup to the strained liquid. Blend everything by hand until you produce a smooth thick sweet sticky liquid or syrup

This syrup worked so well that it was soon commercialized and sold in drugstores up into the 1940's which was when the American Medicinal Association started taking over our lives and pooh-poohing all natural medicine.

On the label of one brand of Yellow Dock Syrup, it read: "This syrup may be taken one teaspoon at a time (As much as 6 times daily) to heal bronchitis and asthma as well as cease tickling or scratching in the throat or the lungs. It can also be taken as a cure for anemia"

The root has of lately been used with positive effect to restrain the inroads made by cancer. Not bad for a lowly common weed! But then, isn't that just like God?

Canaigre, Red Dock or Tanners Dock (Rumex hymenosepalus)

This plant is found all over the Southwest desert wherever a little water collects. Like Yellow Dock, it is used for a pot herb by boiling the young leaves in a few changes of water to remove the taste of the tannins. The roots of this plant are very fat and round and resemble yams. They are sliced and dried for later use as tea or for tincturing.

An infusion of the stems and leaves can be used as a wash for sores, ant bites and infected cuts much the same way you use Yellow Dock.

However there is a big difference in the action of this root on the bowels. Just as its cousin, Yellow Dock, is used for constipation, the roots of this plant are used for even the most stubborn cases of diarrhea. An infusion of the roots or a few teaspoons of the tincture is effective for this. This powerful astringent action is due to as much as 30 percent tannin found in the roots. Because of this super high tannin level, Canaigre is made into one of the best solutions for tanning hides and is still used today for this by many tanners. This is another reason it was always known as a useful cowboy's herb.

The roots are very astringent and taste very bitter and sour causing a very strong reaction in the saliva glands when in contact with the tongue or mouth. An infusion of the roots has been used as a gargle to treat coughs and sore throats. The root has been chewed for the successful treatment of coughs and colds.

The dried, powdered roots are also used as a dusting powder and dressing much the same way you would use Yellow Dock Root powder.

However please remember: the root of Canaigre is used internally to stop diarrhea while the root of Yellow Dock is used internally as a laxative for constipation. You do not want to get these plants mixed up in their internal uses!

Osha Root, Chuchupate or "Bear Medicine" (Ligusticum Porteri)

This is a powerful and legendary herbal medicine. The use of Osha Root was adopted from both the Native Americans and the Mexicans by the early cowboys and was often a part of the wise camp cook/doctor's medicine supply, (In tincture form and sometimes raw dried roots) Although there was not a real knowledge of viruses and bacteria at the time, it was proven over and over that it could cure many types of flu as fast as overnight if caught early! This was a real blessing to the hard working cowboys often exposed to the rain and cold and harsh working conditions.

In modern times Osha has been proven to have a strong anti viral action and can cure many viral infections, even Herpes Zoster (Shingles) and should be tried first for almost any virus. Osha is a very important part of a special formula we created for "Plant Cures Inc" called Viral Defense. It uses 5 other herbs which are Chinese "heat clearing" herbs. This formula continues to be the biggest selling item at Plant Cures simply because it works so well to quickly destroy flu and many other infections. (Viral and bacterial)

During the 1918 flu epidemic the Arapaho Indians were on record as having a cure for this radical flu and they were never sick from this flu for long. (Where as many other Indian tribes suffered many deaths from this flu) It is also on record that they had cured many white people as well. This was accomplished by simply chewing and swallowing dried Osha Roots. The few old medical books that recorded this have mostly all been burned or destroyed as this was quite an embarrassment to the medical system.

This herb is very important to me personally because it saved me (Possibly from death) and cured me of a very stubborn viral pneumonia. In fact it was my healing through the use of Osha Root that caused me to become a clinical herbalist. Please allow me to explain:

I never smoked cigarettes but I was a working musician (working in smoke filled bars) from very early in my life. I am sure this contributed to the aggressive form of Viral Pneumonia I had. This problem would reoccur often. There was a secondary bacterial infection that always seemed to develop so the doctors gave me large doses of penicillin. This would stop it for awhile but it would always return with a vengeance!

My immune system was getting very compromised. It was so compromised that I once caught Chicken Pox for the second time at the age of 35. (This is not supposed to happen) And I caught it from my own son who was only 3 years old at the time!

Once a doctor I saw while traveling said, *"we don't have much we can do for the virus and you are going to lose your immune system entirely if we keep giving you this much penicillin. I am not supposed to say this but have you ever looked into medicinal plants? Some have great anti viral actions. You can find out how to get them in medicinal herb books but if you tell anyone I said this I will have to deny it"*

I almost thought he was nuts but I picked up a medicinal herb book on Southwestern plants. I found a picture of the plant called "Osha" which grows at high altitudes (Often above 10,000 ft.) so I set out to find it in the high mountains near by me here in Arizona. I was blessed and found it the first day! I was so excited I started chewing the roots driving back down from the mountain.

I chewed these strange hot tasting roots every day for about two weeks when I noticed I was completely cured! I could breathe great and the Pneumonia never came back. (It has been over 30 years) After my healing I was just plain hooked on healing with medicinal plants! I got my hand on every book I could find on the subject. I became a pretty darn good botanist. After that I studied hard and got my Master Herbalist degree. From there I went on to study Traditional Chinese Herbal medicine for a TCM degree. But back to Osha!

Interesting facts about Osha: The common Mexican name for the Osha plant is chuchupate. This is actually an ancient Aztec term meaning "bear medicine." Bears respond to the herb like cats do to catnip. They will roll on it and cover themselves with its scent. Males have been seen to dig up the roots and offer them to females as part of courting.

When a bear first comes out of hibernation, it will eat Osha if it can find it, to cleanse it's digestive system. The bear will chew the root into a watery paste, then spit it on its paws and wash its face with the herb. It will then spray the herb over its body as the herb possesses strong action against bodily parasites.

It is not known how the bears came to acquire this herbal knowledge, but their use is legendary in all cultures that refer to it as "bear medicine". This is the reason that the bear is considered to be the prime healing animal in many cultures because it uses plants for its own healing. Any plant that is considered to be "bear medicine" is a potent and primary one.

Osha was originally used by Native Americans to treat colds, flu, and upper respiratory infections. Since Osha displays a strong affinity for the respiratory system, Native American runners would chew the root to increase endurance.

It was also worn in medicine pouches and around the ankles to ward off rattlesnakes. This is a lot more than "Indian superstition" as rattle snakes do not like to get near Osha root for some reason.

Osha is related to lovage and a member of the Parsley family, it is a perennial, growing above 8,000 feet throughout the entire Rocky Mountain range from Mexico to Canada.

The plant stands about two or three feet in height and possesses the characteristic umbel (umbrella) flower shape and leaves that look a little like parsley. It can be stubborn and strong, often growing in aspen groves among their roots, making digging very difficult.

It is one of the few herbs that can be dried in the sun without harm and will last for years in the dried form. It will not rot or mold because of the potent antibacterial and antiviral substances in the root prevent it from doing so.

Desert Tea, Cowboy Tea or "Mormon Tea"

This is a branched broom-like shrub growing up to 10 feet tall, with slender, jointed stems. The leaves resemble large pine needles. Small male and female flowers, blooming in March and April, are borne on these plants in cone like structures. The flowers are followed by small brown to black seeds.

Early pioneers and cowboys were often offered a beverage made from this plant by friendly Indian tribes of the Southwest as a form of hospitality. These pioneers and cowboys found this tea to be not only delicious but discovered that it was very effective for the symptoms of allergy related asthma and that it often helped with urinary tract infections.

The dark brown resinous scales found around the flower buds contained at least one third pure tannin and its powder made an excellent external haemostatic for stopping bleeding from wounds.

In the Southwest this plant was so common that you could find it most anywhere on the trail. However camp cooks always stopped to pick up the greenest and healthiest plants as it stored very well for future use. Sometimes the cook took the small, hard, brown seeds and ground them to be used as a bitter meal or added to bread dough to flavor it.

As a beverage, a small handful of green or dry stems and leaves were placed in boiling water for each cup of tea. It was removed from the fire and allowed to steep for twenty minutes or more until it became dark brown in color.

Going on the fact that this plant could cure urinary tract infections, early doctors tried using a very strong tea of the plant for the treatment of syphilis and other venereal disease. It turned out to be very effective. It soon became standard fare in the waiting rooms of many brothels in early Nevada and California.

History claims it was first introduced to the brothels for using against venereal disease by a Mormon man who frequented a brothel called Katie's Place in Elko, Nevada during the mining rush of the 19th century. This would likely explain the reason it is often called "Mormon Tea"

Although this plant is not as potent as its commercial relative in China, called Ma Huang, this southwestern species contains enough ephedrine-related alkaloid ingredients to make it functional but without the central nervous system stimulation properties that can make Ma Huang dangerous to some. This is why Desert Tea is the perfect safe and effective medicine for allergies and asthma. The isolated drug ephedrine is a strong stimulant and has an effect on the body similar to adrenaline. (Ephedrine is also only one chemical step away from amphetamine)

I have personally used this plant to successfully stop a spring time "hay fever" type allergy that used to plague me every spring here in Arizona. I would drink a cup once or twice a day from early spring to late summer getting amazing relief. However when the next season came around I did not get the allergy reaction at all. It has been many years now and It has never returned.

Goldenseal - Hydrastis Canadensis *(Cherokee name:* Da lo ni gei*)*

Goldenseal root has been used for centuries by the Cherokee Indians for a variety of problems, including healing cuts and wounds, improving appetite, relieving liver and stomach problems, repelling insects (mixed with bear grease), and treating "watery eyes" (probably allergies). Early medical reports show the Cherokee used golden seal to successfully cure external and even some internal cancers as well.

Goldenseal was more of a medical doctor's "drug" in the early 1800's than something the camp cook would carry. However cowboys based in Tennessee, Arkansas, Georgia, and North Carolina often carried the powdered herb and their own homemade *Tincture of Golden Seal* after acquiring the root from local Cherokees. (The Cherokee lived in Tennessee and Arkansas long before the colonists moved in and took over their lands)

By the late 1800's, after word of its powerful healing properties was out, Goldenseal was carried by many camp cooks all over. It became so popular they could even order it by catalog and have it sent anywhere in the country.

Golden seal relieves gingivitis and pyorrhea and, when combined with bicarbonate of soda, makes an excellent mouthwash for healing sores in the mouth and gums. Bicarbonate of soda or "baking soda" is something the camp cook always carried.

From early times all the way up to today Goldenseal remains one of the most scientifically researched herbs of all time. This is simply because modern science has seen it work and work very well for so many diverse things.

Today I believe it should be in anyone's medicine cabinet as it could save so many trips to the doctor that would wind up just harming your immune system from antibiotics.

Here is an extensive list of things research has proven about Goldenseal:

Golden seal increases the secretion of digestive enzymes and fluids, especially bile, which helps regulate liver and spleen functions. Golden seal also reduces inflammation and pain in mucosal tissues, and acts as a laxative. However, golden seal is not recommended for extended periods, (More than a month) because it can reduce the digestive system's ability to absorb some nutrients, especially B vitamins.

Golden seal is recommended for numerous gastrointestinal disorders, including colitis, enteritis, gastritis, hemorrhoids, hepatitis, intestinal infections, and peptic ulcers.

Golden seal acts as an astringent, producing a vaso-constricting—tightening of the blood vessels—effect. This action is due to the presence of an isoquinoline alkaloid called hydrastine, which also stimulates the autonomic nervous system. Golden seal's astringent ability enables it to help tone mucus membranes, which in turn, aids ear, eye, nose and throat problems, stomach and intestinal disorders, prostate and vaginal complaints, and stops internal bleeding and prevents hemorrhaging.

Golden seal helps tighten the tiny capillaries which can cause "red eyes" when the eyes are irritated, and is known to greatly

soothe eye inflammation and treat eye infections, particularly ca-
tarrhal and follicular conjunctivitis. Golden seal acts as a mild
decongestant, relieves excess mucus, and reduces fever and inflammation associated with glandular swelling and sinusitis.

Many doctors have recommended golden seal for treating ulcers
in the uterus and vagina, as well as for gynecological problems such
as dysmenorrhea, menorrhagia, pelvic inflammatory disease, post-
partum hemorrhage and yeast infections. Another isoquinoline alkaloid in golden seal is canadine, which acts as a uterine stimulant.

Golden seal has been shown to help heal damaged tissues resulting from acne, eczema, rashes, smallpox, and other sores or
wounds. Golden seal is often used to treat herpes outbreaks, especially in the genital area (herpes simplex virus II).

Berberine, an isoquinoline alkaloid found in golden seal, has
been studied at length in both clinical and experimental environ-
ments for its antibacterial and amebicidal properties. Berberine
has been shown to have a vast array of antibiotic effects, including
activity against bacteria, protozoa, and fungi, including Candida
albicans. In fact, berberine's antibiotic effect against some of
these pathogens has been shown to be stronger than that of many
commonly-used prescription antibiotics. Furthermore, berberine
possesses the ability to prevent bacteria and yeast overgrowth, a
common side effect of pharmaceutical antibiotics.

Berberine is extremely effective against diarrhea which is
often found in cases of chronic candidiasis. Clinical studies have
documented positive results using berberine with amebiasis, chol-
era, giardiasis and other cases of acute gastrointestinal infection,

including E. coli, Klebsiella, Salmonella, and Shigella. Berberine also exhibits a sedating action on the central nervous system.

Golden seal has been found to potentate insulin and have a hypoglycemic effect which is beneficial for diabetics. Thus, herbalists do not commonly recommend golden seal to individuals with hypoglycemia.

Golden seal is believed to have a long-term effect (2 months) on intestinal flora. Individuals may wish to rotate golden seal with a "friendly" bacteria supplement such as Lactobacillus acidophilus.

Golden seal is high in vitamin C and trace minerals including cobalt, iron, magnesium, manganese, silicon and zinc. Golden seal also contains vitamins A, E, and the B-complex, as well as calcium and potassium.

Women should avoid the use of berberine-containing plants during pregnancy, including barberry, golden seal, and Oregon grape. Individuals with hypoglycemia (low blood sugar) should avoid using golden seal as it lowers blood sugar levels.

Echinacea, "Kansas Snake Root" (Cherokee name: Gv ne ge tsun vs ta)

Few realize it was, once again, the Cherokee who brought this amazing herb to our attention. It is mentioned here just after Golden Seal because the two herbs (Golden Seal and Echinacea combined) is one of the "two herb formulas" that the Cherokees used in their medicine system as a standard for both snake bite and any kind of cold or respiratory problem.

Most "official" herbal formulas in the Cherokee medicine system consist of either two herbs or of seven herbs. (I am not quite sure why) The Cherokee medicine system is closely guarded in its workings and is still fully used today in the Cherokee Nation as one of the best systems in the world. It is integrated into their modern hospitals. Even though these hospitals are fully functioning in normal allopathic western medicine, the Cherokee Plant Elders are always on call.

However this formula is one they shared with the white settlers many years ago. The combo of Golden Seal and Echinacea was given to us mostly as a remedy for poisonous snake bites but it was told that it could cure most any cold or flu type disease contacted along our network of wagon trails.

Also, It was known that the Cherokee used Echinacea extensively to assist with health issues among tribe members. The Cherokee referred to Echinacea as Gv ne ge tsun vs ta.

Cherokee children used the flower and stem in games. The children would hit the stems together; wrapping the stems and meshing the flower heads together which was much like what we know as "Velcro" in its affect of sticking together.

Echinacea is now considered one of the best-known, extremely safe and efficient herbal medicines in use today. This humble annual herb has been shown to fight bronchitis, colds, flu, infection, strep throat, and other immune and respiratory problems. It is a known fact that taking Echinacea at the first sign of cold or flu can arrest the problem and shorten the duration of symptoms.

The mechanism by which Echinacea strengthens immune function to counter bacterial and viral infection is remarkable.

Echinacea contains polysaccharides which resemble bacteria, causing the immune system to regard them as foreign invaders. In turn, the immune system builds up its defenses against Echinacea, increasing the body's production of white blood cells, thereby becoming stronger and more capable of fighting a real bacterial invasion. Even after exposure to a virus, Echinacea can block virus receptors on the surface of cells, preventing the virus from "taking hold." Echinacea also normalizes body temperature, whether high or low.

Echinacea polysaccharides also produce an anti-hyaluronidase effect—the ability to protect hyaluronic acid from being dissolved by a foreign enzyme. Hyaluronic acid forms a protective gel around cells to prevent viral penetration. In addition, Echinacea contains a caffeic acid ester called Echinacoside, which functions as a natural antibiotic, enabling the herb to fight and even prevent infection in much the same way as penicillin.

Furthermore, Echinacea contains fat-soluble substances called alkylamides which provide additional antibacterial and antifungal activity, as well as mild anesthetic effects.

Researchers have also confirmed Echinacea's ability to increase the immune system's production of interferon—the substance which fights viral infections in the body—as well as it's ability to increase production of T-lymphocytes (T-cells) and other white blood cells which fight bacterial toxins. In fact, scientists at the University of Munich found Echinacea stimulates infection-fighting T-cells more than 30% in comparison to other pharmaceutical immune stimulants including synthetic interferon.

Bloodroot Sanguinaria canadendis

Bloodroot was used by the Cherokee and most all eastern Indian tribes as both a red dye and as a very strong medicine. As far back as 1612, Captain John Smith noted in, Jamestown, Virginia, *"They use the bloodroot for swellings, aches, anointing their joints, painting their heads and garments."* He also added that *"they set a partially nude woman fresh painted red"* to entertain the colonists"

Internally it was used (In very small doses of 1-5 drops of the tincture) for coughing and bleeding of the lungs. It was also employed as an expectorant for acute and chronic respiratory tract affections, laryngitis, sore throat, asthma with cold thick phlegm, and croup. It is used effectively in pneumonia by taking only 2-3 drops at a time throughout the day.

It can be added to a cough syrup made of cherry bark, eucalyptus and honey and used for all the above very effectively. A few drops of the tincture was often dropped on a sugar cube and sucked on as a cough remedy. It can be used for adenoid infections, nasal polyps, syphilitic troubles and piles (For piles, they would use a "tea" of bloodroot as an enema)

Small doses stimulate the digestive organs and heart. Large doses act as a sedative and narcotic. The Cherokee Plant Elders advise that when the condition is not easily overcome, combine Bloodroot with equal parts of Goldenseal Root.

Externally, Bloodroot has a very pronounced effect on the skin. The tincture is directly applied for the treatment of fungus, eczema, cancers, tumors, and other skin disorders. It is a good remedy for athlete's foot and rashes. An ointment of bloodroot alone or in combination with other herbs is directly applied to venereal sores, tinea capitis, eczema, ringworm, scabies, and warts. (For warts, it mostly affects those that are cancerous) An ointment was made by mixing an ounce of the powdered root in 3 oz. of lard, bringing t he mixture to a boil, simmering briefly, and then straining.

This all shows Bloodroot as an extremely valuable medicine. However when it comes to cancer, Bloodroot is perhaps the most misunderstood and controversial herb in the history of medicine.

If you do a search on Bloodroot you will always find (Often for sale) the mention of "Black Salves" used to remove skin cancers and even deep underlying tumors. PLEASE DO NOT USE THEM! These salves are made of a mixture of Bloodroot and very caustic Chloride of Zinc. (This is the stuff used in dry cell flashlight batteries) This "remedy" has been used since the early 1800's and many people have been severely disfigured by it.

Under an experienced doctor's care, some may have been able to use this successfully with minimal damage but it was quite dangerous. (Remember this was also the time when people were dying like rats from the doctor's mercury treatments which were used for many different things including syphilis)

Because of these "Black Salves" with their extremely dangerous caustic effect Bloodroot is immediately associated with these and thought of as a dangerous "caustic herb" when nothing could be farther from the truth. (There is an ever-so slight caustic action in bloodroot but nothing at all compared to Chloride of Zinc) The pharmaceutical and cancer industry are delighted with this situation because it keeps people from seriously considering the use of Bloodroot as a remedy for cancer.

The only caustic effect of bloodroot is that it has a very slight die-off effect of cells on the surface that are already beginning to die naturally and a very pronounced effect of killing cells that have become corrupt. This is exactly why it is used for skin cancers. One of the ways this was done was by mixing bloodroot tincture with a little slippery elm powder making a paste and applying it to the problem. They would cover it up with a bandage if necessary and change twice daily. Skin cancers had been reported to be gone in 2-3 days.

Much research has been done on the use of Bloodroot for cancer. Chemists have identified the isoquinoline alkaloids sanguinarine and berberine, (Also found in Golden Seal Root) among others, and an extract, sanguinaria, which shows powerful anticancer activities.

A remarkable series of studies was done by The American Association for Cancer Research. The studies were on Bloodroot (Sanguinaria canadendis) as an anti-cancer substance. If you put the following title into a Google search on your computer you can see these studies at full length. Just put in: *Response of Sanguinarine for Cancer Cells versus Normal Cells*

However, even with these remarkable studies, it is my opinion that the Cancer Industry would never welcome a proven natural cure like Bloodroot for cancer for two reasons:

#1: If it is natural that means you could not get a patent on the drug and no pharmaceutical company could ever profit from it.
#2: If anything that was natural and readily available could cure various cancers (and I personally believe there are lots of things that can) became known to the public, then billions of dollars in research money would cease and huge corporations would fail and many people would be out of work.

"Essiac" A Formula From The Ojibwa (Chippewa) Indians

The formula which I prefer to call "Ojibwa Tea" was made famous by a nurse from Canada named Rene Caisse. She first leaned of it from a patient in the 1920's who said she was completely healed of breast cancer, 20 years earlier, using this formula. (Plus Bloodroot) The patient remembered the herbs and how to identify and collect them exactly as an elderly Ojibwa man had taught her.

She was nice enough to show Rene how to gather the herbs as well. You would have thought that Rene would have been grateful to the woman for showing her this formula and maybe even named the formula after her or at least after the Ojibwa Indians for giving it to her.

However Rene, fancying herself as the "discoverer" of this formula, named it "Essiac" This was her name (Caisse) spelled backswords.

I always refer to this formula as Ojibwa Tea and try to forget about Rene Caisse's "Essiac". None the less this formula is probably now best known as "Essiac Tea"

Another reason I don't refer to this formula as "Essiac" is because the doctor that Rene Caisse worked very closely with in promoting this was Charles Brush. Dr. Brush was also JFKs personal doctor that became known as "Dr. Feel Good". He was called this because he had a reputation for prescribing any drugs you wanted that would make you "feel good" (For a price of course)

However with all this aside this Ojibwa formula turns out to be an extremely good formula for detoxifying and can work well in removing heavy metals from the body. It has also actually helped stop many documented cases of cancer.

The four herbs in this formula are as follows:

Burdock Root

This is used traditionally to help reduce mucus, maintain a healthy gastrointestinal tract, stimulate a healthy immune response, for weak digestion, as a diuretic for waster retention and to sweat out toxins through the skin. It has vitamin A and selenium to help reduce free radicals and its chromium content helps maintain normal blood sugar levels.

As far as its use in the Ojibwa detox tea it functions to stimulate digestion via stimulating a liver action that assists in applying the other herbs action on the body. It also prepares the liver to work at optimum for excreting the chemicals that will help expel unwanted toxins and for optimum liver function in every way.

Sheep Sorrel

Sheep sorrel is a rich source of oxalic acid, sodium, potassium, iron, manganese, phosphorous, beta-carotene, and vitamin C. The combination of these vitamins and minerals promote the glandular health of the entire body. Sheep Sorrell also contains carotenoids and chlorophyll, as well as citric, malic, tannic and tartaric acids. There are also a lot of chemical structures that we will never recognize in this plant.

The chlorophyll can serve many functions in the body. For one, it carries oxygen throughout the bloodstream. This is significant because cancer cells cannot live in the presence of oxygen. Chlorophyll closely resembles hemoglobin in its functioning: both are capable of carrying oxygen to every cell of the organism. When chlorophyll molecules carry oxygen through the bloodstream chromosome, damage can be inhibited to effectively block cancer. Chlorophyll also helps block germs and harmful bacteria.

Sheep sorrel was considered the most active herb for stimulating cellular regeneration, detoxification and cleansing in the formula.

Rhubarb Root

Used traditionally in small amounts, this herb acts as a gentle laxative and helps purge the liver of toxic buildup and waste. It helps neutralize acids due to indigestion. Its malic acid also carries oxygen to all parts of the body, aiding in healing and promoting a positive and balancing effect upon the whole digestive system.

Slippery Elm (Inner bark)

This contains large amounts of tannins and mucilage which help dissolve mucus deposits in tissue, glands and nerve channels. The inner bark, rich in calcium, magnesium and vitamins (A,B,C,K), helps to nourish and soothe organs, tissues and mucus membranes and is helpful to the lungs. It also helps neutralize acids from occasional indigestion. In this formula it would soften the inner lining of the colon making it very easy for the other herbs to remove toxins.

Applications:

My wife and I take a cup of this "Ojibwa Tea" formula two times daily for two weeks in the early spring and two weeks in the fall each year. It helps to remove metal toxins that always seem to get into the body. This metallic toxin is most likely from the Stratospheric Aerosol Geo-engineering (Persistent contrails or "chemtrails") that have been sprayed so heavily here in Arizona.

The Ojibwa would use this formula as an underlining formula for almost any aliment as it was so good for detoxifying the blood. For cancer they also would make a separate "tea" from Bloodroot. This was quite strong so you could only take one mouthful and wait about a half hour. If you did not regurgitate then you took another. This went on until you did regurgitate. This was a bit rough but they claimed it dissolved many tumors in the body using it this way.

When we make this formula at Plant Cures we use 2 oz of Burdock, 2 oz Sheep Sorrel, ½ oz Rhubarb Root and about ¼ oz slippery Elm bark. This is enough for a weeks supply so we ship 4 bags of this out as a months supply. To prepare it, boil it in a gallon of water for 20 minutes and let it set overnight. Next day strain it and put it in a gallon jar (Or two ½ gallon jars) and keep in the refrigerator. Drink a full cup twice daily on an empty stomach.

Dandelion

This is another one of those plants that was often freshly available on the cowboy trails. For food, the young greens provided salads and a great pot herb as well. But this was also such a treasure to use as medicine fresh out of Gods green Earth as well.

The fresh juice of Dandelion is applied externally to fight bacteria and help heal wounds. The plant has an antibacterial action, inhibiting the growth of Staphococcus aureus, pneumococci, meningococci, Bacillus dysenteriae, B. typhi, C. diphtheriae, proteus.

The latex contained in the plant sap was used to remove corns and warts very successfully. All one needed to do was break the fresh stem and use the milky substance inside brushing it on where needed.

Even though the use of this plant was fairly common knowledge from all cultures including the white man's European ancestry, all Indian tribes, and even Chinese Medicine it does not mean that this lowly little weed is any less than an absolute all time hero of all natural medicine! It should get some kind of award!

I find it very ironic and very symbolic when you watch all those lawn weed killing commercials on TV. It is always those poor little dandelions that are being destroyed. The facts are this is almost the only medicine that could save your live from exposure to those same herbicides they are advertising by its amazing ability to detoxify your liver.

As internal medicine, the roots, flowers and leaves were used for different things

As a tonic, Dandelion root strengthens the liver. An infusion (Strong boiled Tea) of the root encourages the steady elimination of toxins from the liver and thereby the whole body. Dandelion is traditionally used as a blood purifier, for constipation, inflammatory skin conditions, joint pain, eczema and liver dysfunction, including liver conditions such as hepatitis and jaundice. I have seen this work well in acute alcohol poisoning where the skin was almost all one big rash.

The roots were often dried and roasted and saved on the trail for being boiled as a coffee substitute when they ran out of the real stuff. It did not taste to bad (A little like coffee if you use your imagination) and it gave you a little "lift" as your liver always got toned up a bit after drinking it. There were probably quite a few cases of hepatitis and other liver related diseases that were avoided from drinking this while the cowboys were saying, *"I'm getting tired of this stuff, I wish we had some real coffee.*

Dandelion (Whole plant – leaves and root) is used for the treatment of the gall bladder, kidney and urinary disorders, gallstones, jaundice, cirrhosis, hypoglycemia, dyspepsia with constipation, edema associated with high blood pressure and heart weakness, chronic joint and skin complaints, gout, eczema and acne.

The leaves of Dandelion are used as a powerful diuretic. (Boiled as a strong tea or in the form of a tincture) This use of this as a diuretic is amazing because although it causes your kidneys to throw off extra water from the body, it still does not deplete the body of potassium.

Research is revealing that the many constituents of Dandelion including Taraxacin, Taraxacoside, Inulin, Phenolic acids, Sesquiterpene lactones, Triterpenes, Coumarins, Catortenoids and Minerals, mainly Potassium and Calcium, are very valuable in curing a number of disorders and illnesses.

The fresh yellow flowers of the plant have a very good effect on the eyesight. (A large part of this is due to a reaction that takes place in the liver) A tincture can be made or the fresh flowers or they can be boiled as a tea. This can be very helpful for those that can not see when first coming in out of the bright light. It is also helpful for many other eyesight problems and should be tried for any of them including certain types of cataracts.

The Cherokee knew of the Dandelion's powerful effect on eyesight and used these flowers for being able to hunt or even in war maneuvers or whenever it was necessary to see in the dark of night.

All these amazing medicinal uses from that pesky little weed that people love to kill when it is found in their lawns.

I personally hold Dandelion with its leaves that are named for lion's teeth, as one of the most curative herbs I know of. At Plant Cures we make a powerful detoxifying kit called "Protox" from Dandelion with a few other herbs including Yellow Dock , Chaparral and Burdock.

The Healing Power of Traditional Chinese Herbal Medicine

The true root of TCM (Traditional Chinese Medicine) goes back about 4,000 years to the Taoists (Not a religious group but a group of philosophers) who came up with the theory of Yin and Yang, The Five Elements and a flow of life in our bodies they called Qi. (pronounced chee) They also discovered and mapped out the body's meridians that this Qi flows through.

However (and most importantly) with the discovery of Yin and Yang, The Five Elements and the "Qi" with its meridians, these wise men REASONED that there had to be a loving creator of all these things (The One who holds Yin an Yang and every-thing in the universe together) They called this creator The Sheng Di which translates into "Heavenly Father/Creator." Remember these Taoists did not have a religion, or any false "god". They were just "thinkers". No they certainly did not know Jesus (This was 4,000 years ago anyway) but I find it amazing that they actually REASONED that there had to be a loving creator. These were truly wise men. By the way, please remember to pray for China, many people are becoming Bible believing Christians there (In spite of their government) at a remarkable rate.

The Discovery of Yin and Yang and the Five Elements

Yin and Yang are the symbols of opposing energies with Yin being cold, dark, small, compressed, watery, and shy as directly apposed to the opposite Yang being hot, bright, large, expanding, fiery and aggressive. These examples are of the extreme end of things. In other words if there was a little cold to cool down the hot or a little hot to warm up the cold it would be more desirable than just hot or cold. So it was noted that finding a perfect balance of Yin and Yang in all things leads to a more balanced peaceful place, especially within the balance of our bodies.

Then these wise men looked very closely at what the basic elements of creation were. They defined these five elements of God's creation as water, wood, fire, earth and metal. They discovered that these elements play an important part of discovering the nature of our internal organs, how they relate to these elements, and how our bodies go on living and reproducing cells.

Each of these basic elements like everything under the sun is subject to Yin and Yang (they can be hot or cold, dry or wet etc.) Also, each of these five elements in Traditional Chinese Medicine relates to different organ systems within our bodies.

Here's how it breaks down:

Water: This element represents the kidneys, bladder, Reproductive system, and all fluids other than blood in the body.

Wood: This element represents the liver and gall bladder.

Fire: This element represents the heart, pericardium, blood and the "triple burner", (the three areas of heated distribution of water)

Earth: This element represents the stomach and spleen (digestion and metabolism)

Metal: This element represents the lungs and colon.

The Discovery of the Energy Flow called "QI" and its Meridians

These wise men also discovered the amazing life flow in us (and all God's living creation). They called this flow of energy, "Qi", (Pronounced Chee) I personally believe this is witness of the breath of life that God breathed into us. They discovered that this "Qi" flows throughout the body in currents or conduits or what we now call channels or meridians. In Chinese this meridian system is called the Jing Luo.

Within the Jing Luo there are fourteen main channels and along these channels "entry points" were discovered that mapped out the very same acupuncture points we use today in many of our modern hospitals. Twelve of these channels connect to the twelve corresponding internal organs from which each meridian derives its name.

For example, the wood element's yin organ is the liver. The liver channel runs from the foot (Between the big toe and the next) up the inside of the leg, along the center of one-half of the abdomen and goes inside below the sixth rib. Inside it connects to the liver and the gallbladder, goes up through the diaphragm, up to the throat, then the eyes and terminates at the vertex of the skull. There are two branches from the liver channel; one which connects to the inside of the lips and one which connects with the lung.

Exactly how they discovered these channels is a bit of a mystery. We know that they did not cut into bodies. They would never expose the eternal organs which they considered "The heavenly jewels". Most feel that these Taoist's were so sensitive they could feel the energy under the skin with precise direction. Some of the early anatomy drawings for books were based on this and they were surprisingly accurate.

How Traditional Chinese Medicine Works:

This discovery of Yin and Yang the five elements, the flow of Qi and how they all relate to our body became the root of the most accurate diagnostic tool in the history of medicine! This is known today as the **Five Element Diagnostic System** and it is integrated even into our western medicine system in some hospitals. It is used in all hospitals in China and in a few hospitals in the US and many others around the world.

In very basic terms this system works by finding the Yin or Yang energy imbalances (Hot, Cold, Dry Damp etc.) in each of the major organ systems of the patient. (This is found by the doctor questioning, looking at the tongue, and feeling the pulses) Then the plants and herbs with the exact opposite energies of the patient are applied to bring balance to the patient's whole body. For example if there are heat toxins found in a lot of the body then the appropriate heat clearing herbs are applied. It turns out that these heat clearing herbs were found later to have powerful anti-viral and anti-biotic actions.

However, the TCM doctor never knew that 3,000 years ago and it did not mater at all that he did not. Even today, modern science never really has to enter the picture at all. (Although it is often fun to see the proof that it works)

China may seem like an "evil empire" to us (And in some ways, I guess it is) but we owe so much to them for giving us this wonderful system. Please pray for the Chinese people. They are one of the fastest growing Christian nations in the world even though they have to keep the church "underground". But the facts are these Chinese Christians are willing to risk this for Jesus. And I can tell you they make such wonderful Christians when they get saved!

The Chinese Herbs and Chinese Herbal Formulas

To be fair, the herbs found in the United States are no less remarkable than anywhere else on earth. Even the Chinese will admit that our American Ginseng is in many ways superior to Chinese Ginseng. No place else has Bloodroot, Echinacea, or our amazing Golden Seal Root. God has blessed the whole earth with His incredible healing plants.

It is not so much the herbs that are found in China but the fact that the Chinese have had over 3,000 years of experience using herbs as medicine. They now have over 8,000 medically logged plants in an ongoing system that has continually been practiced since its beginning! They know their weeds to say the least!

I have often wondered what it would have been like if the Chinese had, instead, had America as their source for herbs to use as medicine. I am sure it would have been just as good.

So in the next pages I want to share with you a few of the best Chinese herbs and herbal formulas I have come to know over my 30 years as a TCM herbal practitioner.

Tian Qi; The Herb Chinese Medicine Was Named From

(Pronounced Tin Chee)

Tian Qi is certainly not an herb that was ever found growing out on any American wagon trail. However, we know that the Chinese railroad workers had brought this herb over with them from China and it is on record that the early American doctors of the west were remarkably impressed with the medicinal qualities of this amazing herb.

These early homeopathic and Eclectic Physicians quickly established trade with China for importing this herb. It was this herb along with the Chinese formula called Yin Qiao (Mentioned in the next sub-title) that helped give the Eclectic Doctors the credibility they needed to build 8 accredited Eclectic Medical schools, and 9 Homeopathic schools by 1915. These schools all produced students that sat for the various state boards and took the same tests as everyone else. During this time there were 12,000 Eclectic physicians and 14,000 Homeopathic Physicians in practice. During this time my great grandfather came over from France and became an American

Homeopathic Physician who made much of his own medicine from plants he gathered.

A few camp cooks that kept in touch with these doctors must have carried this herb due to its amazing use for traumatic injuries. Also it is a known fact from records and early photos that many of these camp cooks were, in fact, Chinese themselves. These Chinese camp cooks were hired for their talents as both cooks and their reputation as Herbal Doctors. The cowboys highly respected these Chinese Camp Cooks.

Tian Qi is at the top of the list of medicinal herbs in the Chinese Herbal Medicine system containing over 8,000 logged medicinal herbs. It is the root of the plant that is used and it is very dense and heavy. (I have broken machines from grinding it) It is used mostly in powdered form but sometimes a tincture is used.

This herb used to be a part of the original ideogram symbolizing the word for "Chinese Medicine" about 3,000 years ago. The ideogram portrayed a farmer beating a snake with a hoe and a snake escaping by going into a hole and winding itself around a root.

This Chinese ideogram tells the story of the farmer that kept finding a large snake in his garden. He tried to kill it by chopping it with his hoe. After the snake was quite torn up and left for dead the farmer would see the same snake return a few days later perfectly healed.

One day he followed the snake to see what it was doing. He found the snake would borough into the ground and wind himself around the roots of Tian Qi. It would stay there for a few days until it was healed and then re-emerge. This story became the symbol of Chinese Herbal Medicine. It was later (Sometime in the 1800's) replaced by an ideogram that shows a wine flask and a plant which is symbolizing an herbal tincture but personally I liked the old one best.

My personal experiences with Tian QI

These four following "case histories" had nothing to do with ANY of my patients but had everything to do with ME and my own misfortunes! And I promise you, nothing is made up here (I wish it was!), I only hope I don't get the "privilege" of having any more personal reasons to brag about the amazing healing powers of this herb.

Please always remember though, if you have broken bones, let a doctor set them for you before you begin herbal treatments. This is one of the few good things doctors still do when they are not busy pushing dangerous drugs!

Case 1:

Shortly after I got my first practice together as a Clinical Master Herbalist I made some good friends out in China Town, S.F. and established some very good Chinese bulk herb trading. Suddenly I had everything that I studied about over the last few years at my finger tips and not a moment too soon!

I didn't have many patients yet so I had some time do a little upkeep around our little ranch. We have a chicken coop made out of that old style corrugated steel that a lot of roofs are made out of and I thought those poor chickens could use another window.

After marking the window space I started cutting it with a jig saw. Things were going fine until I heard the whistling sound of an Arizona dust devil right behind me. There were quite a bit of big metal shavings from the jig saw all over the freshly exposed window ledge. The twister picked them up and fired them at me like a machine gun! I felt something go into my eye.

It didn't hurt all that much at first and I figured it would just wash it self out so I finished the window hole and went in the house to check on my eye.

I got one of those magnifying mirrors and a magnifying glass to look at my eye and I saw this little "spike" with about a quarter of an inch of it sticking out from the middle of my eye. It was located right in the cornea.

Tweezers were the first thing I tried but the metal must have been barbed from the cutting. It just kind of stretched my eye as I pulled and man did it hurt! I thought about just yanking it out fast but I realized I might pull a bit of my eye out with it and besides I almost stabbed my eye with those tweezers the first time!

Next, I tried a magnet since it was steel and that hurt worse with no luck getting it out.

Suddenly I remembered all the lessons and stories I heard about raw Tian QI powder and how the Chinese used this for many kinds of injuries. Mostly it is used to direct the blood, stop bleeding without clotting, and yet speed up blood flow where it is needed. All this while helping stop pain. Almost, I thought, like it had a healing desire of its own.

I remembered hearing how it is still issued to Asian soldiers today for stopping bleeding from bullet wounds. Also I had heard that in many cases it somehow could pull or push or "float" the bullet to the surface due to the "directing" of blood from this herb.

I hadn't seen a western doctor in 10 years or more and I wasn't going to start my new herbal practice off by going to one now!

I decided to use some raw Tian Qi powder and boil it in water until I had a nice warm "gooey" substance and placed it into my eye. I then covered my eye with a stick-on bandage and decided to go to bed and see what happened in the morning.

When I woke up the bandage had fallen off and I could not open my eye. It was cemented together by the Tian Qi that had dried like glue on the outside of my eye. It was as hard as a rock. I put some hot water on it until it softened and I could feel my eye start to open. Then I realized I had crunchy dried pieces of Tian Qi inside my eye. I washed them out with a cloth and got the old magnifying mirror out and looked at my eye. Praise God, The spike was gone. I looked at the rag with the crunchy stuff on it and there was a little metal spike with a definite nasty looking barbed edge!

If I had gone to a hospital it would have to have been surgically removed along with a not so small piece of my eye. However, the floating, moving, and directing action of the Tian Qi gently some how "wiggled" the barbed steel out of there.

My eye felt great and I was prouder than I could be of that Chinese Tian Qi root and my God who created it.

Case 2:

Only a few weeks later I was building some rustic Southwestern furniture in my shop (which was what I did for a living before I became an herbalist) I was ripping some old barn-wood boards on my table saw and apparently I had missed removing an old nail out of one of them. Suddenly, something hit me in the middle of the forehead and knocked me to my knees! I thought someone had just shot me in the head! I became unconscious for a few seconds and when I got up there was a quite a stream of blood running down me. I came in the house and almost scared my wife to death!

We washed everything out and didn't see any piece of nail in my head but it just did not want to stop bleeding. I covered the hole with Tian Qi powder and the bleeding stopped almost immediately. I also drank a little Tian Qi "tea" as I thought this would help with the pain (I really had a nasty headache!) and also I thought it would speed up the healing. I soon felt only a tingling numbness in my head with very little pain.

The next day it had not clotted over but yet the bleeding had stopped and there was only a light pink bit of fluid around the wound so I thought I would wash it out and put some more Tian Qi on it. As I was washing it I heard something metallic hit the tile floor. I looked down and it was not a nail at all. It was a large tooth from the saw blade that broke off from hitting the nail and had hit me like a bullet! The saw blade had been turning at about 10,000 RPMs so it hit me at the speed of a bullet. My head healed without a scar. and I don't think I even got any "Drain Bammage" but one is never sure!

Case 3:

I don't know why but I guess I have always been a little accident prone. Also somebody said things happen a lot in threes! Well this next incident happened about a year later when I was again at the table saw. I was ripping some boards for more shelving for my herbal supply this time!

It was getting a little dark and I had not turned the lights on yet but I only had one more shelf to make so I cut it. After the cut, I reached down to move a piece of debris from the saw table and stuck my left thumb right into the spinning saw blade! It knocked me back against the wall and when I looked at my thumb, the top part of it (half way to the first knuckle) was just hanging by a thin piece of skin.

I held my thumb back in place, walked into the house and once again I about scared my wife to death. However she was getting a little used to it by now.

I thought about how Tian Qi has a way of "directing" blood flow and that if I just put a lot of Tian Qi powder between my two thumb pieces and some how could "weld" or "cement" something around my thumb to hold it in place it would grow back together. I decided that Comfrey root powder mixed with vodka was the perfect cement. (It is almost like rubber glue) In my practice, I used to call this "Liquid Stitches" and had used it to heal and hold deep cuts together on animals and humans. It would dry soon so I covered my thumb with it and made a kind of protective brace with two sticks and some tape and went to bed.

The next morning it was leather hard around my thumb and it didn't hurt all that much. Later that day it dried much harder and since the "comfrey cement" was all the way around my thumb it started to cut my circulation off a bit so I peeled it off slowly to change it. I noticed that my thumb sections were already netting together so I put more Tian Qi around the raw areas and cement-ed around it again with the Comfrey glue or "Liquid Stitches". I kept this up for about one week. It healed beautifully.

There is only a slight dent in my thumb now and it is just a little shorter than the other one since a little "meat" was taken off the thumb from the saw. My thumbnail was never lost and I have good feeling in my thumb except for a tiny bit of tingling in spots when I touch it just right.

I always wondered what an emergency room doctor would have done. Would I still have my entire thumb? I don't think so.

Case 4

Well, this last case just happened only a few months ago as of this writing! (Just for all you wonderful readers I guess) Keep in mind; this is about twenty years after "case 3"

I was using a chain saw to cut a bunch of Nopalitas cactus "trees" at the trunks that had died from a hard winter freeze. The trunks were hard in most places but had a few rotten soft places in them as well. I was cutting on one that was up against a brick wall so I had to make the cut come towards me away from the wall…… Well you guessed it. I hit a soft spot in the cactus and the chain (running at full speed) came straight through into my left leg just above my knee.

It was a perfect hit! It left about a 4 inch long by half inch deep by half inch wide open gash. I limped quietly into the house and asked my wife if she could go to the office for me and bring back some Tian Qi powder. She actually kept very calm and asked, "So what did you do this time?" I told her and she came back with the Tian Qi in about one minute.

I took of my pants and was sitting there in my shorts while watching it bleed pretty fast. When I poured the Tian Qi powder into the wound, it stopped bleeding immediately. Just then a cowboy friend of ours who was working on our fence line walked in. He saw me with blood still all over my leg and asked if I needed him to take me to the hospital. My wife just laughed and said, "Oh, you don't want to ask Chris that" We all just sat around laughing (What else can you do?) and I realized at that time that I was no longer in any pain.

Just a few minnutes later a friend drove up on his tractor to help us smooth out our dirt driveway. I had washed the blood off by then and went out in my shorts to help direct the job. (OK, I guess I was in a bit of mild shock) He never knew anything had happened until I told him about a half hour later when we went into the house.

I started thinking about all the possible infection between the rotten cactus and the filthy chain saw blade so I washed out the Tian Qi and poured a teaspoon or so of our liquid Viral Defense (A blend of antiviral and antibiotic herbs tinctured in alcohol) into the wound. Now that hurt! Wow! It really hurt! I poured some more Tian Qi into the wound and it quit hurting.

For about two weeks I changed the wound alternating with Viral Defense and Tian Qi. I watched as slowly the flesh filled in where about a half inch deep, half inch wide 4 inch long, gash used to be. It took a only few weeks.

No I never saw a doctor, no I never applied any stitches and yes I was able to mount my horse by myself in about two weeks. (This it what I had prayed for – I was not quite sure what I had cut through in my leg)

Today there is just a nice pretty pink straight looking scar and all is well with the world. Nothing hurts or even tingles. Once again, thank you God for being the great healer and thank you for that Tian Qi Root! I only have one request: **Please don't let me have to write case # 5, Lord!**

Other Common Uses of Tian Qi

Tien Qi root (Panax Pseudo-Ginseng) in a raw fine powdered form is carried by most Asian soldiers as standard military issue. It is carried in a small bottle for pouring into an open wound or for taking internally if necessary.

The reason this is standard issue is its amazing ability to "redirect" the blood from an open wound and even helps push or "float" metal objects to the surface. It can literally help stop bleeding without necessarily clotting. However, it can aid in clotting if it is necessary. It's almost as if it has a mind of its own. The Chinese say it "disciplines the blood"; also when taken internally, it can really speed up the healing time of wounds, broken bones, or most any tissue damage.

Tien Qi powder is taken internally for many reasons such as healing from an operation, wounds, internal bleeding and broken bones. This is also 100% applicable to female problems of severe menstrual bleeding and is used commonly by women in China. Tien Qi is very effective for this.

About ¼ to ½ teaspoon of the powder dissolved in hot water or tea is taken 2-3 times a day for internal use. When I take it I have always noticed a nice warm energy coming from the stomach area and also found that when I take it, I am very alert and more focused than usual. This is most likely due to the added movement and "discipline" of the blood around the brain area.

Tien Qi is also used in a very famous Chinese liniment called Zhang Gu Shui to facilitate healing of broken bones and sprains due to its ability to disperse blood from an injury. It will stop bruises and other hematoma quickly by this dispersion. The exact formula is "kept secret" but everyone knows that the main herb is Tien Qi in a menthol-camphor base. (The Menthol Camphor helps carry the herb deep into the tissue.)

I used to practice the martial arts (Kung Fu) and there was always a bottle of Zheng Gu Shui around at all the tournaments in case someone was injured. I have heard countless stories of major Karate tournaments in China where someone's leg had been broken fighting so they wrapped the leg, putting cotton balls soaked in Zheng Gu Shui or another very similar formula under the wrap and sent him back to fight! (and he won)

Yin Qiao (Yin Qiao Jie Du Wan) The Honeysuckle and Forsythia Pill

This formula originally appeared in Wen Bing Tiao Bian (Detailed Analysis of Seasonal Febrile Diseases, 1798 A.D.) by Wu Tang. It was primarily used, In Chinese terms, to clear heat toxins and to release the exterior of the body for the treatment of wind-heat affliction with chills and fever, headache, and sore throat. In western terms, this means it is **literally a cure for the common cold**. And guess what! It works and works fast. I have seen it cure colds overnight or just in a few days many times.

The formula is composed of Forsythia (Lian qiao), Lonicera flower (which is the common Gold and Silver Honeysuckle known as Jin yin hua), Platycodon Root(Jie geng), Herba Mentha (Bo he), Prepared soybean (Dan dou chi), Bamboo leaf (Zhu ye), Licorice (Gan cao), Schizonepeta spike (Jing jie sui) and Arctium fruit (Niu bang zi).

In America, it was introduced by the Chinese railroad workers to many people and quickly caught the attention of common doctors. It is believed that this formula, as well as Tien Qi, (Mentioned above) were the two Chinese Medicines responsible for the Eclectic Physicians being formed and becoming so popular starting in the 1840's.

This was the kind of fast working, easy to take "Miracle Medicine" that made what the common doctors had at the time look absolutely worthless in comparison. The Eclectics were already proving there was much better medicine around with the use of Native American herbal remedies and it was the addition of formulas like this (From the other side of the world) that helped to coin the phrase "Eclectic Doctors".

I am sure that many of the traveling salesmen with their "Medicine Shows" got a lot of return customers from this formula. And I am also sure that many of our early traditional cowboys and camp cooks took advantage of this.

Yin Qiao is regarded as highly effective for treating common cold, influenza, certain acute disorders, mainly onset of infection and inflammation, marked by sore throat, congestion, feverish feeling, and aching in the muscles. This remedy is famous in China, and is the most commonly used herbal remedy of Chinese families today.

Our own family has always had this around and it has never failed us. It is always available at Plant Cures and is a big selling "return customer" item. We have personally passed out a lot of this as gifts to friends. After they get rid of a cold in two days (that usually takes two weeks to go away) it changes their whole way of thinking about medicine, sneaky huh?

Bi Yan Pian "Open Nose Tablet"

This herbal formula has been around for many years and is traditionally used for respiratory allergies and even asthma with chronic ongoing lung infections or upper trachea infections that are some how related to allergies. It is very effective for that cedar pollen stuff people suffer from in the Hill Country of Texas and works for just about any form of respiratory allergy from just about anything.

I have seen this work when there are un-explained respiratory problems that doctors wind up prescribing dangerous steroid inhalers for. It is a crime how the doctors push these steroids and ruin people's long term health just because the FDA approves it!

When Bi Yan Pian is taken with Desert Tea. (Seen earlier in this chapter as "Desert Tea, Cowboy Tea or Mormon Tea") The two can be an effective combo to totally heal someone from a nagging asthma type respiratory problem that they may have had for years. (If infection is a major player a heat clearing formula like Viral Defense should be added to the mix) The Desert Tea is what cured me of a nagging "every summer – all summer" allergy thing I had for most of my life. I used the Bi Yan Pian for relief when things got bad and I wound up having to use it less and less as time went on. Next summer it never came back. I have had no problem for over 25 years now.

Some of the things I hear a lot of from Bi Yan Pian users are: "It's so good to be able to taste my food again!" - "I quit having to take my allergy pills!" - "You don't know how much energy I have now that I can breathe again" - "What? There are no drugs in this?"

The list of Chinese herbs in this are Xanthium sibiricum fruit, Magnolia denudata flower, Forsythia suspensa fruit, Ledebouriella divaricata root, Angelica dahurica root, Anemarrhena asphodeloides rhizome, Glycyrrhiza uralensis root, Schizonepeta tenuifolia herb, Chrysanthemum indicum flower, Schisandra chinensis fruit, Platycodon grandiflorum root. The Chinese names for these herbs are: Cang er zi, Xin yi hua, Lian qiao, Fang feng, Bai zhi, Zhi mu, Gan cao, Jing jie, Ye ju hua, Wu wei zi, Jie geng.

Bu Zhong Yi Q Wan or "The Central Qi Pill"

There are so many (thousands actually) of very effective traditional Chinese patent herbal formulas that a large book could be written on them so I certainly can't list them all here. However, another outstanding formula that truly should be mentioned here is Bu Zhong Yi Qi Wan often called the "Central Qi Pill"

The Ingredients in Bu Zhong Yi Qi Wan are Astragalus membranaceus root, Glycyrrhiza uralensis root, Codonopsis pilosula root, Atractylodes macrocephala rhizome, Angelica sinensis root, Cimicifuga foetida rhizome, Bupleurum chinense root, Citrus reticulata peel, Ziziphus jujuba fruit, Zingiber officinale rhizome-fresh. The Chinese names for these herbs are: Huang qi, Gan cao, Dang shen, Bai zhu, Dang gui, Sheng ma, Chai hu, Chen pi, Da zao, Sheng jiang

The TCM system has long recognized a very close connection between the digestion (In this case meaning the absorption of nutrients into the blood via the stomach-spleen system) and the response of the nerves, muscles and connective tissue.

When this system is addressed with the right group of herbs to support the "qi" or energy which flows through this system, a remarkable healing process is started. This is very effective on problems relating to muscles as well as problems relating to digestion. I have personally seen this "Central Qi" formula help in a very big way (If not completely cure) with all of the problems mentioned below -both digestive and muscular.

For digestive problems, this formula has been effective for gastric prolepses, hemorrhoids, hiatal hernia, chronic colitis, ulcerative colitis, Crohn's disease, celiac disease, and chronic hepatitis.

For muscle problems it is used for muscle atrophy, fribromyalgia, muscles that have been stretched abruptly or torn and even multiple sclerosis and much more!

A very good indicator that this formula will help you out is a look at the tongue. When one needs this formula, the tongue can look pale with very prominent teeth marks showing. (These teeth impressions will show up on the sides of the tongue where it rests on the teeth) This indicates the muscles (Which the tongue is a perfect model of) are lacking in Qi and do not firm-up as they should. A TCM practitioner may also notice the pulse will often feel deficient and rootless at the Stomach/Spleen position on the right hand.

So many people complain sometimes of "just being sore all over" or noticing that they groan a lot when getting up from a chair. They should try Central Qi. The nice thing is with formulas like this you can always try it with out worrying about any bad effects. And this is a formula that will most likely help with any muscle discomfort or digestive problem so you can see why I just had to mention it in this book.

Dan Shen: The Amazing Heart Normalizing Blood-Red Sage Root

Salvia miltiorrhiza; Radix

My teacher at The University Of Arizona Medical Center was Dr. Wen Zi. He was, a 12th generation Chinese Herbal Doctor in China and with dual citizenship he was a Western MD Cardiologist. (Head of Cardiology at the U of A Medical Center) He could not say enough about this amazing herb known as Dan Shen!

In China, Dr. Zi had seen Dan Shen work in a wide variety of coronary diseases replacing dangerous pharmaceutical drugs and correcting the problem beautifully.

Many official clinical tests have taken place in China and many other countries. Most testing in the cases of angina showed close to 90% of those tested were significantly helped! About 80% of arrhythmias were corrected or at least improved. And in many cases, the valves of the heart have actually shown to have been helped over long term use correcting many problems.

If you are suffering from any heart disorder I can most definatly recommend trying Dan Shen. If you are on any heart drugs, and want to get off them, now is the time! some may have to "wean" off of them slowly (1-3 weeks) before or as you start using this herb due to an addiction reaction to the drug. (However drugs can throw off the way herbs work many times - Just cowboy up and don't do drugs is the best thing I can say!)

Also if you are on Coumadin or other blood thinners be advised that you will **not** need it when taking Dan Shen as Dan Shen will also thin the blood.(But not at all in the same toxic way! Dan Shen keeps your blood at optimum health!) Get off of the Coumadin or, if you must, be sure to have your blood checked.

BUT REMEMBER! there are two different "target test numbers" – One for "normal healthy people not taking Warfarin and one target for those taking this poison or other "blood thinners" and if they have ever prescribed it to you once, you will always be on the "taking Warfarin" list as they just can't accept that you might refuse to take it.

If you quit taking your "blood thinner" and they don't know you have (Or don't accept the fact that you have) then your blood (according to these idiot doctors) would have to be 2.0 – 3.0 to be healthy. Yet for a "normal healthy person" (with the common sense to not have ever taken this poison in the first place) the normal range would be 1.5 -2.0! So of course your blood would appear thicker when you quit taking Warfarin even if is totally normal and even better than it was! Are we confused yet? Trust me that is exactly what they want! Anything to keep you on this drug! Doctors are brainwashed on this and it is almost 100% of them that just can't see it any other way. It is truly amazing.

He Shou Wu and other Superior Tonic Herbs

In Traditional Chinese Medicine, there are over 8,000 logged and fully understood (In their energy factors) official medical herbs used in thousands of formulas. However there is also a small grouping of herbs called The Superior Herbs. Out of over 8,000 herbs only about sixty belong to this classification. These are the true tonic herbs associated with longevity. Although everyone is different in their balances of Yin, Yang, Chi, Jing, Shen, Blood, Heat, Moisture, and other factors, This group of Superior Herbs are those herbs that can benefit just about anyone.

These Superior Tonic Herbs are not considered to be 'medicinal' in the usual sense of the word. They are not used to treat specific diseases or disorders, yet such things as weak sore knees, poor eyesight, low sexual energy, impotence and infertility, high blood pressure, high cholesterol, obesity, general week vitality, even gray hair, and many other things that plague many of us are often completely cured by these Superior Tonic Herbs.

Remember these symptoms (just mentioned above) are the ones most commonly treated by doctors with the <u>most deadly</u> of all pharmaceuticals. This is why I have always said doctors should concentrate on traumatic injuries and stay far, far away from our God given natural balance of health with their "Science" and Pharmaceuticals.

Out of these 60 Superior Tonic Herbs, I would have to say that He Shou Wu (Polygonum multiflorum) is, to me, the most amazing tonic of all with longevity being the key factor. . It is widely used in Chinese herbal medicine as a tonic to prevent premature aging by tonifying the Kidney and Liver functions. It also is known to bring up Jing (vital essence), nourishing the blood, and fortifying the muscles, tendons and bones. It strengthens and stabilizes the lower back and knees. He Shou Wu can also increase sperm count in men, even in old age. It helps build ova in women as well making it quite useful for fertility.

Weak painful knees are another sign of kidney deficiency as is lower back pain and low sexual energy. He Shou Wu is quite often the answer! I personally started taking He Shou Wu on a daily basis as my knees would hurt when I would walk up or down stairs. After only about a week of taking this the pain in my knees just went away and I could run up and down stairs like a kid again.

I have been taking He Shou Wu on a daily basis now for about 8 years as of this writing and will take it the rest of my life if I can still maintain a trusted herb trade with China. (This worries me a bit but if I can no longer import this herb I will start taking our American Chaparral Herb as a "tea" in small doses every day as a replacement)

He Shou wu works good in raw powder (A heaping teaspoon once daily) or extract powder in capsules (3-5 capsules twice daily) or the tincture (1 teaspoon twice daily) I take it mostly in raw powder form. A big heaping teaspoon in the morning mixed in a smoothie or sometimes just in organic chocolate milk. Sometimes I also take the tincture at night as it makes for a good sleep. (Yet when I take it in the morning it energizes me)

He Shou Wu is widely used in Asia to maintain the youthful condition and color of the hair. This is, for some reason, it's most popular attribute but it does so much more than this! However there are a whole host of more important health benefits surrounding this incredible tonic herb.

There are countless stories of people that have lived well past the century mark taking this herb, including Li Qing Yeun who lived to be an amazing 197 years old! (The longest living person in recent history) Li collected wild herbs and sold them for a living most of his life. His death in 1933 was reported in the New York Times and many other major newspapers. However "science" tries to deny this and tell you that the longest living person was a lady in France that reached 124 in spite of the well documented history of Li Qing Yeun. There are many distortions from the Chinese government that even claim Li Qing Yeun lived to the age of 256 but I personally think that is hogwash – He claimed he was 197 – Why would he lie and claim he was 197 if he had lived to the age of 256? Was he embarrassed by his old age? (Give me a break)

He Shou Wu is prepared traditionally in China by slicing the root shortly after harvesting and then cooking it in black bean soup (in a proportion of 10 parts He Shou Wu to 1 part black beans) until the soup is exhausted. The "prepared" roots are then dried. This process has been done in this way for around 1,500 years. If the herb is not prepared in this way it will not have the same tonic energy. However raw un-treated He Shou Wu is often used in formulas to stop acne and also for its strong laxative effect.

He Shou Wu is a tonic for the endocrine glands; it improves health, stamina and resistance to disease. It is used to reduce cholesterol because of its lecithin. It is used for angina pectoris, bloody stools, hypoglycemia, diabetes, night sweating, schizophrenia, chronic bronchitis, epilepsy, head injuries, impotence, malaria, sores, cuts, and ringworm. It promotes red blood cells, helps rid intestinal parasites, and is good for resistance to cold.

Science has actually taken the study of this plant very seriously as there were way too many cases of true longevity associated with this herb to ignore. The studies showed that He Shou Wu improves the cardiovascular system, enhances immune functions, slows the degeneration of glands, increases antioxidant activity, and reduces the accumulation of lipid peroxidation.

Such findings suggest that He Shou Wu is helpful in combating some of the processes that lead to the conditions and characteristic of old age, thereby also reducing the risk of fatal diseases (e.g., cancer) and incidents such as heart attack, stroke. He Shou Wu was shown to have effects on the antioxidant system superoxide dismutase (SOD), accumulation of lipid peroxidase, and enhancement of cell-mediated immune responses.

These were very important findings and were promptly "swept under the rug" by the main stream medical system.

Studies have also demonstrated that various laboratory animals fed He Shou Wu in their diets lived longer than control animals: A decoction with He Shou Wu as the main ingredient prolonged the life span of fruit flies. At 0.1% strength, the decoction could prolong the lifespan by 5.83%. At 0.5% strength, it could prolong the lifespan by 12.03%.

He Shou Wu has been shown to slow down the aging of vital organs in aged animals, especially the reproductive organs, the ovary, the uterus and the testicle. The same formula also demonstrated significant results in open human clinical studies.

In an attempt to prove Shou Wu's legendary reputation as being able to reverse grey hair to black, Shou Wu liquor (dilute alcohol extract) was given to 36 people with premature gray hair. 24 completely recovered their dark hair and 8 more showed improvement. The total effective rate was 88.9%.

As for me and my hair it did not do quite that much (I guess I could not be considered prematurely gray) but it did take it from a ghostly white to a darker gray with even a few flecks of brown and black. (My original color) The main thing is my knees and much of my body does not hurt now and I feel so much younger than I used to. That is something I praise God for!

Tying it all together:

An entire book with over a two thousand pages could be written on the many herbs and their medical applications I just don't want to be the one to write it. However there are many great books on Chinese Herbal Medicine and American medicinal herb uses out there. If this interests you in a big way (And I sincerely hope it does) please go to your closest big city libraries and check out as many books as you can on this. A very good and easy to read book on Chinese herbs I can recommend is *Chinese Herbal Medicine* by Daniel P Reid. (This is a sort of soft cover "coffee table" book with lots of illustrations)

We desperately need more people with a true working knowledge of medicinal plants. We need more and more real natural thinking "cowboy herb doctors" Remember it was these wonderful people of long ago that helped form the great Eclectic Physicians Colleges that ALMOST caught on. We could have had a naturally based great medical system in this country had it not been for the newly formed Boston AMA taking their cue from the newly formed FDA.

We don't need a bunch of "NEWTS" (Remember, that's *New Experts With Ties)* We don't need these "geniuses" telling everyone how great they are with plant medicine because they were educated beyond their intelligence by someone connected with the medical system. Scientists and doctors are the last ones anyone should listen to when it comes to using herbs as medicine.

And please remember, **we would seldom even need medicinal herbs** if we really put nutrition on the front burner of our lives.

To re-cap here are a few things to remember if you want to live a non chemical, nutritionally sound life. These will help you reap the benefits of seldom getting sick from anything as well as adding many years to your life on earth:

Stay away from margarine of any kind; Use only real butter.

Never use anything but raw organic sugar or honey as a sweetener. None of the artificial sweeteners are safe and you will NOT lose any weight by using them.

Always use only sea salt or natural pink salt.

*Refuse anything (even water) that was ever warmed or cooked in a microwave oven. **This is very important!***

Make sure most everything you eat is certified organic or grown or raised by yourself with absolutely no herbicides, pesticides, or inorganic fertilizers. Be very careful of chicken, if it does not say Certified Organic, chicken is extremely dangerous. (It is sometimes packed in formaldehyde) Also Stay away from any and all "fast food" (Especially those chicken nuggets and any thing with "Mc" attached to its name)

Do not eat anything that is GMO (Genetically modified organism) produced. If it does not say Certified Organic then all corn, wheat, soy and most any grain you eat is most likely GMO.

***And here is the real biggie that will be hard for many folks: Don't do prescription drugs!** Learn how to replace everything with good solid herbal medicine. (Your doctor will disown you but so what) Also don't even do isolated vitamins, or isolated "health products" like CO Q 10. Just get what you need from whole plants, herbs, natural whole minerals and the natural whole food that you eat.*

The hardest thing to overcome is that which is blatantly pushed in our faces as "truth". However it is actually a lie from the pit of hell. This is the work of the media, who is controlled by Satan himself, desperately trying to push poisonous processed foods and deadly deceiving dangerous drugs as the "healthy modern way of life". "Healthcare" is the largest and most deadly genocidal scam that was ever perpetrated. In essence, the following paragraph is exactly what they are telling us:

"Just listen to us and take our drugs, kiddies, we are the experts; God did not know what he was doing when he gave us those "weeds" to use as medicine. Also, don't bother with that hard to prepare, out

of date, whole natural food when we have all these scientifically pre-pared "wonder meals" waiting for you". **I ask you, just who does that sound like???**

How do we know that this is Satan? Simply because these pharmacy products are all based on greed! (And we all know who the author of greed is) These products are designed simply for making money from suckers like the American consumer and with out any regard for our health. In fact, in an attempt to cover their butts, they even tell you how death, cancer, deformities, tu-berculoses, you name it, may be possible if you take what they are pushing. Now here is the big **BUT;** *"But if you ask your doctor if it is right for you, then he will most likely say, YES and everything will magically be OK"*

Now what is legally going on behind this scam is the drug companies figure they are protected because "your doctor" (Who people often so ignorantly put their faith in) would be the one you would have to sue. And there are two factors that the doctor is counting on to protect him. The first is they are so friendly and "nice" and know just what to say, that that you will not likely sue him. The second is these MDs have so much medical insurance that they are prepared for a lawsuit to happen on a regular basis. They just go play golf and let the insurance company handle it. This is almost the perfect crime-partner re-lationship. You **can** sue the drug companies but the expense of battling their lavish lawyer teams is way beyond most people's means.

For one last time, let's look at:

"What would the early American Cowboy say about this?"

"OK, so your saying that although you know this drug could kill me, all I need to do is ask Ol' Doc Mathews about it and if he says, "Yeah, go ahead it's safe", then it will be safe for me to take? Well first of all I did ask Doc Mathews. He just told me I was a fool to listen to people like you with that kind of double talk. Then he said, "What is that Rx thing on that fancy prescription paper?" I looked it up in my new encyclopedia and I found out it means "Take this prescription in the name of Jupiter" - **In the Name of Jupiter?!! What kind of demons has this guy been sleeping with? I know I ain't been to church in a while but even I know to stay away from fellers like that!** *Not only would I say, "Don't take that" but I think we better get hold of Sheriff Baxter real fast! This guy is a killer for sure and he needs to be behind bars".*

Well, as you know these lies about drugs and processed foods are plastered all over the billboards, super markets and magazines. They are also eternally blasted at us on TV and radio. So the question arises, *"Are you going to keep falling for it, or are you going to cowboy up and say NO to all these lies?"*

At the introduction of this book I talked about Christians having discerning. Well something that might help you with having that healthy discerning of what is right before God is coming up right here in the next chapter.

Chapter 5:
Taking God's Ultimate
Medicine;

OK, now you found the keys to perfect health (Well, OK, maybe a little closer to perfect health than you were anyway) but the bible says in Mark 8:36 *"For what shall it profit a man, if he shall gain the whole world, and lose his own soul?"* If you know God wants you as healthy as you can be in this life, what do you think he wants for your eternal life after death?

One thing I know our God doesn't want for you is eternal death and destruction. However in preparing for your life after death, there are no organic foods you can eat that will save you from an otherwise genuine hell, no herbs, no perfect blue sky without any "Chemtrails", no cure. That is, no cure other than the blood that Jesus shed on the cross.

The answer is simply become born again! All you have to do is reach out and take the hand that He has provided. Your sins have already been paid for. They were paid in full on the cross over

2,000 years ago. All you have to do is reach out and accept it with your whole heart.

It is like finding the absolutely perfect "elixir of life" or the "fountain of youth". That "medicine" if you will, is standing right in front of you waiting for you to take it. You can figuratively pour it into a tablespoon and look at it, hold it up to the light and even smell it but it will not do a thing until you take it. So how do we take it?

Just, admit you are a sinner and tell God you know He is the only thing that can cleanse your sin. Then believe with all your heart that Jesus died on the cross and then rose again all for the sinners of this world. This is how you take that medicine! This will save you from an eternity of hell.

To look at this in the direct light of God's word using scriptures from The Holy Bible, here it is:

The Bible says there is only one way to Heaven:

Jesus said: *"I am the way, the truth, and the life: no man cometh unto the Father but by me."* (John 14:6)

Know that good works cannot save you:

"For by grace are ye saved through faith; and that not of yourselves: it is the gift of God: Not of works, lest any man should boast." (Ephesians 2:8-9)

Be willing to turn from sin. (Repent)

Jesus said: *"I tell you, Nay: but, except ye repent, ye shall all likewise perish."* (Luke 13:5)

Believe that Jesus Christ died for you, was buried, and rose from the dead.

"For God so loved the world, that he gave his only begotten Son, that whosoever believeth in him should not perish, but have everlasting life." (John 3:16)

Pray this now (In your own words) and truly mean it in your heart!

Dear God, I am a sinner and need forgiveness. I believe that Jesus Christ shed His precious blood and died for my sin. I am willing to turn from sin. I now invite you, Jesus to come into my heart and life as my personal Savior,

In Closing:

Remember, of course we can't be perfect in our health at all times but the more you get started with it, the easier and easier it becomes. A simple change to eating organic food WILL make a huge difference in the way you feel and the way you appear to others. This could be the spark that ignites the flame to light up a long healthy drug free life for you on earth. It could take that depression that keeps you from thinking you can't do something and change it into, **"With Jesus, I can do anything I put my heart and mind into".** And when you start using herbs as your source of medicine and find yourself not getting sick anymore, a real wakeup light will go on and you will never turn back!

God has wonderful plans for all of us and good health is always in His plan because He included the way to good health as part of His word, creation and plan. Even after chastising us with the breaking down of the Earth's original firmament (which we know as Noah's flood) His had has provided us an easy way to live to the age of around 120

The only problem is most of us became led astray from God's plan of health for us. It was so easy to forget that **His hand really has provided all that we need.** It was always right there in front

153

of our noses but when we got tricked into thinking we needed more convenience in life it caused us to look in an entirely different direction. .

God's hand really did provide us with convenience in so many ways when you think about it! Look at the neat way bananas are "packaged" with their "easy peel wraps" or how about those individual bite sized sections packed into oranges. Picking apples off a tree or reaching up to pick a cherry or reaching down to pick a strawberry and eat it. Now that is really hard work!

God is a lot of things and the one thing I know for sure is that our God is a JUST God. He knew how easy it was going to be for us to slide off the road of His health plan with all the processed food and drugs with the media hype and all.

God does take pity on us and because he does, He gave us this simple three word remedy that we can use anytime we need it. It is simply, "JESUS FORGIVE ME" That is all you have to ask of God, no matter how dark of a situation you are in, or what you did to your health by just being a bit "stupid". (As most of us can relate) If you sincerely ask God to forgive you He will always give you another chance to start clean again.

As Christians, the biggest thing I know of that separates us from the rest of the world is the fact that WE ARE FORGIVEN. So just BE forgiven and start being healthy by letting Him guide your every step. It is really just that simple.

I sincerely hope you enjoyed this book and through it, found ways to come to better health in this life. Thank you all so much for reading this and giving whole natural food and natural herbal medicine a chance. You can always find us at plantcures.com when you need anything in particular in the way of herbs and natural medicine. .

So until we meet again, partner, may God bless you and thanks for "riding along" with me in this book! I hope so very much to, one day, see you in those beautiful eternal trails and green pastures where we can ride along with Jesus himself. Wow! Riding with the Creator of the universe? Now that is something to look forward to. I can't wait to see His horse!

God bless you all!

Chris Gussa

Bibliography

Much of the information in this book is stuff I have known for most of my life so I apologize if I have missed anyone who may have been a resource.

The late Dr. Wen Zi of the University of Arizona Medical Center has been a very big source of my Traditional Chinese Herbal Medicine knowledge.

I would like to thank RFD TV for some of the Cowboy History.

Liza Veith, *The Yellow Emperor's Classic of Internal Medicine*, University of California Press 1984 (Original Manuscript dating back to 2697 BC)

Charles F. Millspaugh *American Medicinal Plants*, Dover Publishing 1974 (originally published in 1892)

J. I. Lighthall, *The Indian Folk Medicine Guide*, Popular Library 1969 (Original text published in 1883)

Joseph Meyer, *Natures Remedies*, Indiana Botanic Gardens 1934

Michael Moore, *Medicinal Plants of the Mountain West*, New Mexico Press 1979

Michael Moore, *Medicinal Plants of the Desert and Canyon West* New Mexico Press 1989

Qu Jingfeng, Zhang Shaohua, Xie Rong, *The Chinese Materia Medica* Publishing House of the Shanghai College of Traditional Chinese Medicine 1990

Henry C. Lu, *Chinese Herbal Cures*, Sterling Publishing 1991

Daniel P Reid , *Chinese Herbal Medicine* Shambala Publications 1996

Time Life Books: *The Cowboys*

James P Carter, *Racketeering In Medicine*, Hampton Roads Publishing 1992

www.geoengineeringwatch.org *Geo Engineering Watch*

www.naturalnews.com *Natural News*, Mike Adams

www.mercola.com, Dr. Joseph Mercola